How the Immune System Works

FOURTH EDITION

Lauren Sompayrac, PhD

WILEY-BLACKWELL

A John Wiley & Sons, Ltd., Publication

This edition first published 2012 © 2012 by John Wiley & Sons, Ltd.

Wiley-Blackwell is an imprint of John Wiley & Sons, formed by the merger of Wiley's global Scientific, Technical and Medical business with Blackwell Publishing.

Registered office: John Wiley & Sons, Ltd, The Atrium, Southern Gate, Chichester, West Sussex, PO19 8SQ, UK

Editorial offices: 9600 Garsington Road, Oxford, OX4 2DQ, UK
The Atrium, Southern Gate, Chichester, West Sussex, PO19 8SQ, UK
111 River Street, Hoboken, NJ 07030-5774, USA

For details of our global editorial offices, for customer services and for information about how to apply for permission to reuse the copyright material in this book please see our website at www.wiley.com/wiley-blackwell.

First published 1999
Second edition 2003
Third edition 2008
Fourth edition 2012

Cover image and Figure 1 used with permission from Lennart Nilsson photography / Boehringer Ingelheim / SCANPIX.

Library of Congress Cataloging-in-Publication Data
Sompayrac, Lauren.
   How the immune system works / Lauren Sompayrac. – 4th ed.
      p. cm.
   Includes bibliographical references and index.
   ISBN 978-0-470-65729-4 (pbk. : alk. paper)   1. Immune system.
   2. Immunity.   I. Title.
   [DNLM: 1. Immune System–physiology.   2. Immune System–anatomy & histology.
3. Immune System–physiopathology.   4. Immunity–physiology. QW 504 S697h 2012]
   QR181.S65 2012
   616.07'9–dc23
                              2011024775

A catalogue record for this book is available from the British Library.

Set in 9.5/13 pt Palatino by Toppan Best-set Premedia Limited
Printed and bound in Malaysia by Vivar Printing Sdn Bhd

2   2013

Contents

Acknowledgments

I would like to thank the following people, whose critical comments on the earlier editions were most helpful: Drs. Mark Dubin, Linda Clayton, Dan Tenen, Jim Cook, Tom Mitchell, Lanny Rosenwasser, and Eric Martz. Thanks also go to Diane Lorenz, who illustrated the first and second editions, and whose wonderful artwork can still be found in this book. Finally, I wish to thank Vicki Sompayrac, whose wise suggestions helped make this book more readable, and whose editing was invaluable in preparing the final manuscript.

How to Use This Book

I wrote *How the Immune System Works* because I couldn't find a book that would give my students an overall view of the immune system. Sure, there are as many good, thick textbooks as a person might have money to buy, but these are crammed with every possible detail. There are also lots of "review books" that are great if you want a summary of what you've already learned – but they won't teach you immunology. What was missing was a short book that tells, in simple language, how the immune system fits together – a book that presents the big picture of the immune system, without the jargon and the details.

How the Immune System Works is written in the form of "lectures," because I want to talk to you directly, just as if we were together in a classroom. Although Lecture 1 is a light-hearted overview, meant to give you a running start at the subject, you'll soon discover that this is not "baby immunology." *How the Immune System Works* is a concept-driven analysis of how the immune system players work together to protect us from disease – and why they do it this way.

In Lectures 2 through 10, I focus more closely on the individual players and their roles. These lectures are short, so you probably can read them all in a couple of afternoons. In fact, **I strongly suggest that you begin by reading quickly through Lectures 1–10.** The whole idea is to get an overall view of the subject, and if you read one lecture a week, that won't happen. Don't "study" these ten lectures your first time through. Don't even

bother with the Thought Questions at the end of each lecture. Just rip through them. Then, once you have a "feel" for the system, go back and spend a bit more time with these same ten lectures to get a clearer understanding of the "hows and whys."

In Lectures 11–14, I discuss the AIDS virus, vaccines, allergies, autoimmune diseases, and cancer. These lectures will let you "practice" what you have learned in the earlier lectures by examining real-world examples of the immune system at work. And Lecture 15 – A Critique of the Immune System – will help you put in full perspective just how wonderful the immune defense really is. So after you have gone through Lectures 1–10 twice, I'd suggest you read these last five lectures. When you do, I think you'll be amazed by how much you now understand about the immune system.

In some settings, *How the Immune System Works* will serve as the main text for the immunology section of a larger course. For a semester-long undergraduate or graduate immunology course, your professor may use this book as a companion to a comprehensive textbook. In this situation, reviewing the appropriate lecture in *How the Immune System Works* as your course proceeds will help you keep the big picture in focus as the details are filled in. It's really easy to get lost in the details.

No matter how your professor may choose to use this book, you should keep one important point in mind: I didn't write *How the Immune System Works* for your professor. This book is for you!

The Anytime, Anywhere Textbook

Wiley DESKTOP EDITION

For the first time, your textbook comes with free access to a **Wiley Desktop Edition** – a digital, interactive version of this textbook which you own as soon as you download it.

To view your Wiley Desktop Edition, you need to download and install 'Bookshelf' at **www.vitalsource.com/downloads** to your computer, laptop or mobile device.

Your Wiley Desktop Edition allows you to:

Search: Save time by finding terms and topics instantly in your book, your notes, even your whole library (once you've downloaded more textbooks)

Note and Highlight: Colour code, highlight and make digital notes right in the text so you can find them quickly and easily

Organize: Keep books, notes and class materials organized in folders inside the application

Share: Exchange notes and highlights with friends, classmates and study groups

Upgrade: Your textbook can be transferred when you need to change or upgrade computers

CourseSmart gives your students instant access (via computer or mobile device) to this Wiley-Blackwell eTextbook and its extra electronic functionality, at 40% off the recommended retail print price. See all the benefits at **www.coursesmart.com/students**.

It also offers you an immediate, efficient, and environmentally-friendly way to review this textbook for your course. For more information visit **www.coursesmart.com/instructors**.

With CourseSmart, you can create lecture notes quickly with copy and paste, and share pages and notes with your students. Access your Wiley CourseSmart digital textbook from your computer or mobile device instantly for evaluation, class preparation, and as a teaching tool in the classroom.

Simply sign in at **http://instructors.coursesmart.com/bookshelf** to download your Bookshelf and get started. To request your desk copy, hit 'Request Online Copy' on your search results or book product page.

LECTURE 1

An Overview

Immunology is a difficult subject to study for several reasons. First, there are lots of details, and sometimes these details get in the way of understanding the concepts. To get around this problem, we're going to concentrate on the big picture. It will be easy for you to find the details somewhere else. A second difficulty in learning immunology is that there is an exception to every rule. Immunologists love these exceptions, because they give clues as to how the immune system functions. But for now, we're just going to learn the rules. Oh, sure, we'll come upon exceptions from time to time, but we won't dwell on them. Our goal is to examine the immune system, stripped to its essence. The third difficulty in studying immunology is that our knowledge of the immune system is still evolving. As you'll see, there are many unanswered questions, and some of the things that seem true today will be proven false tomorrow. I'll try to give you a feeling for the way things stand now, and from time to time I'll discuss what immunologists speculate may be true. But keep in mind that although I'll try to be straight with you, some of the things I'll tell you will change in the future (maybe even by the time you read this!).

I think the main reason immunology is such a tough subject, however, is that the immune system is a "team effort" that involves many different players interacting with each other. Imagine you're watching a football game on TV, and the camera is isolated on one player, say, the tight end. You see him run at full speed down the field, and then stop. It doesn't seem to make any sense. Later, however, you see the same play on the big screen, and now you understand: that tight end took two defenders with him down the field, leaving the running back uncovered to catch the pass and run for a touchdown. The immune system is just like a football team. It's a network of players who cooperate to get things done, and just looking at one player doesn't make much sense. You need an overall view. That's the purpose of this first lecture, which you might call "turbo immunology." Here, I'm going to take you on a quick tour of the immune system, so you can get a feeling for how it all fits together. Then in the next lectures, we'll go back and take a closer look at the players and their interactions.

PHYSICAL BARRIERS

Our first line of defense against invaders consists of physical barriers, and to cause real trouble, viruses, bacteria, parasites, and fungi must first penetrate these shields. Although we tend to think of our skin as the main barrier, the area covered by our skin is only about two square meters. In contrast, the area covered by the mucous membranes that line our digestive, respiratory, and reproductive tracts measures about 400 square meters – an area about as big as two tennis courts. The main point here is that there is a large perimeter which must be defended.

THE INNATE IMMUNE SYSTEM

Any invader that breaches the physical barrier of skin or mucosa is greeted by the innate immune system – our second line of defense. Immunologists call this system "innate" because it is a defense that all animals just naturally seem to have. Indeed, some of the weapons of the innate immune system have been around for more than 500 million years. Let me give you an example of how this amazing innate system works.

Imagine you are getting out of your hot tub, and as you step onto the deck, you get a large splinter in your big

How the Immune System Works, Fourth Edition. Lauren Sompayrac. © 2012 John Wiley & Sons, Ltd. Published 2012 by John Wiley & Sons, Ltd.

toe. On that splinter are many bacteria, and within a few hours you'll notice (unless you had a lot to drink in that hot tub!) that the area around where the splinter entered is red and swollen. These are indications that your innate immune system has kicked in. In your tissues are roving bands of white blood cells that defend you against attack. To us, tissue looks pretty solid, but that's because we're so big. To a cell, tissue looks somewhat like a sponge with holes through which individual cells can move rather freely. One of the defender cells that is stationed in your tissues is the most famous innate immune system player of them all: the macrophage. If you are a bacterium, a macrophage is the last cell you want to see after your ride on that splinter. Here is an electron micrograph showing a macrophage about to devour a bacterium:

You will notice that this macrophage isn't just waiting until it bumps into the bacterium, purely by chance. No, this macrophage actually has sensed the presence of the bacterium, and is reaching out a "foot" to grab it. But how does a macrophage know that a bacterium is out there? The answer is that macrophages have antennae (receptors) on their surfaces which are tuned to recognize "danger molecules" characteristic of common microbial invaders. For example, the walls that surround bacteria are made up of fats and carbohydrates that normally are not found in the human body. These foreign molecules represent "find me and eat me" signals for macrophages. Indeed, when macrophages detect danger molecules, they begin to crawl toward the microbe which is emitting the foreign molecule.

When it encounters a bacterium, a macrophage first engulfs it in a pouch (vesicle) called a phagosome. This vesicle is then taken inside the macrophage, where it fuses with another vesicle termed a lysosome. Lysosomes contain powerful chemicals and enzymes which can destroy bacteria. In fact, these agents are so destructive that they would kill the macrophage itself if they were

released inside it. That's why they are kept in pouches. Using this clever strategy, the macrophage can destroy an invader without "shooting itself in the foot." This whole process is called phagocytosis, and this series of snapshots shows how it happens:

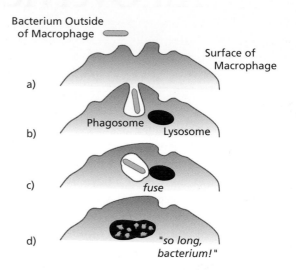

Macrophages have been around for a very long time. In fact, the ingestion technique macrophages employ is simply a refinement of the strategy that amoebas use to feed themselves – and amoebas have roamed the earth for about 2.5 billion years. Why is this creature called a macrophage, you may be wondering. "Macro," of course, means large – and a macrophage is a large cell. Phage comes from a Greek word meaning "to eat." So a macrophage is a big eater. In fact, in addition to defending against invaders, the macrophage functions as a garbage collector. It will eat almost anything. Immunologists take advantage of this appetite by feeding macrophages iron filings. Then, using a small magnet, they can separate macrophages from other cells in a cell mixture. Really!

Where do macrophages come from? Macrophages and all the other blood cells in your body are made in the bone marrow, where they descend from self-renewing cells called stem cells – the cells from which all the blood cells "stem." By self-renewing, I mean that when a stem cell grows and divides into two daughter cells, it does a "one for me, one for you" thing in which some of the daughter cells go back to being stem cells, and some of the daughters go on to become mature blood cells. This strategy of continuous self-renewal insures that there will always be blood stem cells in reserve to carry on the process of making mature blood cells.

As each daughter cell matures, it has to make choices that determine which type of blood cell it will be when it grows up. As you can imagine, these choices are not random, but are carefully controlled to make sure you have enough of each kind of blood cell. For example, some daughter cells become red blood cells, which capture oxygen in the lungs, and transport it to all parts of the body. Indeed, our stem cell "factories" must turn out more than two million new red blood cells each second to replace those lost due to normal wear and tear. Other descendants of a stem cell may become macrophages, neutrophils, or other types of "white" blood cells. Just as white wine really isn't white, these cells aren't ~~~~~~~~~~ They are colorless, but biologists use the ~~~~~~~ ~~~~ lack hemoglobin,

Delete

Red Blood Cell
(Erythrocyte)

When the cells which will mature into macrophages first exit the bone marrow and enter the blood stream, they are called monocytes. All in all you have about two billion of these cells circulating in your blood at any one time. This may seem a little creepy, but you can be very glad they are there. Without them, you'd be in deep trouble. Monocytes remain in the blood for an average of about three days. During this time they travel to the capillaries, which represent the "end of the line" as far as blood vessels go, looking for a crack between the endothelial cells that line the capillaries. These cells are shaped

like shingles, and by sticking a foot between them, a monocyte can leave the blood, enter the tissues, and mature into a macrophage. Once in the tissues, most macrophages just hang out, do their garbage collecting thing, and wait for you to get that splinter so they can do some real work.

When macrophages eat the bacteria on that splinter in your foot, they give off chemicals which increase the flow of blood to the vicinity of the wound. The build-up of blood in this area is what makes your toe red. Some of these chemicals also cause the cells that line the blood vessels to contract, leaving spaces between them so that fluid from the capillaries can leak out into the tissues. It is this fluid which causes the swelling. In addition, chemi~~~~~~ ~~~~~~ased by macrophages can stimulate nerves in the ~~~~~~ that surround the splinter, sending pain signals to ~~~~rain to alert you that something isn't quite right in ~~~~a of your big toe.

~~~~ing their battle with bacteria, macrophages also ~~~~ ice and give off (secrete) proteins called cytokines. ~~~~ are hormone-like messengers which facilitate com~~~~ication between cells of the immune system. Some of ~~~~ytokines alert monocytes and other immune system ~~~~ traveling in nearby capillaries that the battle is on, ~~~~ influence these cells to exit the blood to help fight the ~~~~idly multiplying bacteria. And pretty soon, you have ~~~~igorous "inflammatory" response going on in your toe, ~~~~ the innate immune system battles to eliminate the ~~~~vaders.

When you think about it, this is a great strategy. You have a large perimeter to defend, so you station sentinels (macrophages) to check for invaders. When these sentinels encounter the enemy, they send out signals (cytokines) that recruit more defenders to the site of the battle. The macrophages then do their best to hold off the invaders until reinforcements arrive. Because the innate response involves warriors like macrophages, which are programed to recognize many of the most common invaders, your innate immune system usually responds so quickly that the battle is over in just a few days.

There are other players on the innate team. For example, in addition to the "professional phagocytes" like macrophages, which make it their business to eat invaders, the innate system also includes the complement proteins that can punch holes in bacteria, and natural killer (NK) cells which are able to destroy bacteria, parasites, virus-infected cells, and some cancer cells. We will talk more about the macrophage's innate system teammates in the next lecture.

THE ADAPTIVE IMMUNE SYSTEM

About 99% of all animals get along just fine with only natural barriers and the innate immune system to defend them. However, for vertebrates like us, Mother Nature laid on a third level of defense: the adaptive immune system. This is a defense system that actually can adapt to protect us against almost any invader. It is most likely that the adaptive immune system was designed to protect us and the other vertebrates against viruses, because, as you will see, the innate immune system is not terribly effective against viruses.

One of the first clues that the adaptive immune system existed came back in the 1790s when Edward Jenner began vaccinating the English against smallpox virus. In those days, smallpox was a major health problem. Hundreds of thousands of people died from this disease, and many more were horribly disfigured. What Jenner observed was that milkmaids frequently contracted a disease called cowpox which caused lesions on their hands that looked similar to the sores caused by the smallpox virus. Jenner also noted that milkmaids who had had cowpox almost never got smallpox (which, it turns out, is caused by a close relative of the cowpox virus).

So Jenner decided to conduct a daring experiment. He collected pus from the sores of a milkmaid who had cowpox, and used this to inoculate a little boy named James Phipps. Later, when Phipps was re-inoculated with pus from the sores of a person infected with smallpox, he did not contract that disease. In Latin, the word for cow is *vacca* – which explains where we get the word vaccine. History makes out the hero in this affair to be Edward Jenner, but I think the real hero that day was the young boy. Imagine having this big man approach you with a large needle and a tube full of pus! Although this isn't the sort of thing that could be done today, we can be thankful that Jenner's experiment was a success, because it paved the way for vaccinations that have saved countless lives.

Smallpox virus was not something humans encountered regularly. So Jenner's experiment showed that if the human immune system were given time to prepare, it could produce weapons that could provide protection against an invader which it never had seen before. Importantly, the smallpox vaccination only protected against smallpox or closely related viruses like cowpox. Phipps was still able to get mumps, measles, and the rest. This is one of the hallmarks of the adaptive immune system: It adapts to defend against specific invaders.

Antibodies and B cells

Eventually, immunologists determined that immunity to smallpox was conferred by special proteins that circulated in the blood of immunized individuals. These proteins were named antibodies, and the agent that caused the antibodies to be made was called an antigen – in this case, the cowpox virus. Here's a sketch that shows the prototype antibody, immunoglobulin G (IgG):

As you can see, an IgG antibody molecule is made up of two pairs of two different proteins, the heavy chain (Hc) and the light chain (Lc). Because of this structure, each molecule has two identical "hands" (Fab regions) that can bind to antigens. Proteins are the ideal molecules to use for constructing antibodies that can grasp attackers, because different proteins can fold up into a myriad of complex shapes.

IgG makes up about 75% of the antibodies in the blood, but there are four other classes of antibodies: IgA, IgD, IgE, and IgM. All of these antibodies are produced by "B cells" – white blood cells that are born in the bone marrow, and which can mature to become antibody factories called plasma B cells.

In addition to having hands that can bind to an antigen, an antibody molecule also has a constant region (Fc) "tail" which can bind to receptors (Fc receptors) on the surface of cells like macrophages. In fact, it is the special structure of the antibody Fc region that determines its class (e.g., IgG vs. IgA), which immune system cells it will bind to, and how it will function.

The hands of each antibody bind to a specific antigen (e.g., a protein on the surface of the smallpox virus), so in order to have antibodies available that can bind to many different antigens, many different antibody molecules are required. Now, if we want antibodies to protect us from every possible invader (and we do!), how many different antibodies would we need? Well, immunologists have made rough estimates that about 100 million should do the trick. Since each antigen binding region of an anti-body is composed of a heavy chain and a light chain, we could mix and match about 10 000 different heavy chains and 10 000 different light chains to get the 100 million different antibodies we need. However, human cells only have about 25 000 genes in all, so if each heavy or light chain protein were encoded by a different gene, most of the B cell's genetic information would be used up just to make antibodies. You see the problem.

Generating antibody diversity by modular design

The riddle of how B cells could produce the 100 million different antibodies required to protect us was solved in 1977 by Susumu Tonegawa, who received the Nobel Prize for his discovery. When Tonegawa started working on this problem, the dogma was that the DNA in every cell in the body was the same. This made perfect sense, because after an egg is fertilized, the DNA in the egg is copied. These copies are then passed down to the daughter cells, where they are copied again, and passed down to their daughters, and so on. Therefore, barring errors in copying, each of our cells should end up with the same DNA as the original, fertilized egg. Tonegawa, however, hypothesized that although this is probably true in general, there might be exceptions. His idea was that all of our B cells might start out with the same DNA, but that as these cells mature, the DNA that makes up the anti-body genes might change – and these changes might be enough to generate the 100 million different antibodies we need.

Tonegawa decided to test this hypothesis by comparing the DNA sequence of the light chain from a mature B cell with the DNA sequence of the light chain from an immature B cell. Sure enough, he found that they were different, and that they were different in a very interesting way. What Tonegawa and others discovered was that the mature antibody genes are made by modular design.

In every B cell, on the chromosomes that encode the antibody heavy chain, there are multiple copies of four types of DNA modules (gene segments) called V, D, J, and C. Each copy of a given module is slightly different from the other copies of that module. For example, in humans there are about 40 different V segments, about 25 different D segments, six different J segments, and so on. To assemble a mature heavy chain gene, each B cell chooses (more or less at random) one of each kind of segment and pastes them together like this:

You have seen this kind of mix-and-match strategy used before to create diversity. For example, 20 different amino acids are mixed and matched to create the huge number of different proteins that our cells produce. And to create genetic diversity, the chromosomes you inherited from your mother and father are mixed and matched to make the set of chromosomes that goes into your egg or sperm cells. Once Mother Nature gets a good idea, she uses it over and over – and modular design is one of her very best ideas.

The DNA that encodes the light chain of the antibody molecule is also assembled by picking gene segments and pasting them together. Because there are so many different gene segments that can be mixed and matched, this scheme can be used to create about 10 million different antibodies – not quite enough. So, to make things even more diverse, when the gene segments are joined together, additional DNA bases are added or deleted. When this "junctional diversity" is included, there is no problem creating 100 million B cells, each with the ability to make a different antibody. The magic of this scheme is that by using modular design and junctional diversity, only a small amount of genetic information is required to create incredible antibody diversity.

Clonal selection

In the human bloodstream, there is a total of about three billion B cells. This seems like a lot, but if there are 100 million different kinds of B cells (to produce the 100 million different kinds of antibodies we need for protection), this means that, on average, there will only be about thirty B cells in the blood that can produce an antibody which will bind to a given antigen (e.g., a protein on the surface of a virus). Said another way, although we have B cells in our arsenal that can deal with essentially any invader, we don't have a lot of any one kind of B cell. As a result, when we are attacked, more of the appropriate B cells must be made. Indeed, B cells are made "on demand." But how does the immune system know which B cells to make more of? The solution to this problem is one of the most elegant in all of immunology: the principal of clonal selection.

After B cells do their mix-and-match thing and paste together the modules required to form the complete recipes for their heavy and light chain antibody proteins, a relatively small number of these proteins is made – a "test batch" of antibody molecules, if you will. These tester antibodies, called B cell receptors (BCRs), are transported to the surface of the B cell and are tethered there with their antigen binding regions facing out. Although each B cell has roughly 100 000 BCRs anchored on its surface, all the BCRs on a given B cell recognize the same antigen.

The B cell receptors on the surface of a B cell act like "bait," and what they are "fishing for" is the molecule which their Fab regions have the right shape to grasp – their "cognate" antigen. Sadly, the vast majority of B cells fish in vain. For example, most of us will never be infected with the SARS virus or the AIDS virus, so our B cells which could make antibodies that recognize these viruses never will find their match. It must be very frustrating for most B cells. They fish all their lives, and never catch anything!

On occasion, however, a B cell does make a catch. When a B cell's receptors bind to its cognate antigen, that B cell is triggered to double in size and divide into two daughter cells – a process immunologists call proliferation. Both daughter cells then double in size and divide to produce a total of four cells, and so forth. Each cycle of cell growth and division takes about 12 hours to complete, and this period of proliferation usually lasts about a week. At the end of this time, a "clone" of roughly 20 000 identical B cells will have been produced, all of which have receptors on their surface that can recognize the same antigen. Now there are enough to mount a real defense.

After the selected B cells proliferate to form this large clone, most of them begin to make antibodies in earnest. The antibodies produced by these selected B cells are slightly different from the antibody molecules displayed on their surface in that there is no "anchor" to attach them to the B cell's surface. As a result, these antibodies are transported out of the B cell and into the bloodstream. One B cell, working at full capacity, can pump out about 2000 antibody molecules per second! After making this heroic effort, most of these B cells die, having worked for only about a week as antibody factories.

When you think about it, this is a marvelous strategy. First, because they employ modular design, B cells use relatively few genes to create enough different antibody molecules to recognize any possible invader. Second, B cells are made on demand. So instead of filling up our bodies with a huge number of B cells which may never be used, we begin with a relatively small number of B cells, and then select the particular B cells that will be useful against the "invader du jour." Once selected, the B cells proliferate rapidly to produce a large clone of B cells whose antibodies are guaranteed to be useful against the invader. Third, after the clone of B cells has grown sufficiently large, most of these cells become antibody factories which manufacture huge quantities of the very antibodies that are right to defend against the invader. Finally, when the invader has been conquered, most of the B cells die. As a result, we don't fill up with B cells that are appropriate to defend against yesterday's invader, but which would be useless against the enemy that attacks us tomorrow. I love this system!

What antibodies do

Interestingly, although antibodies are very important in the defense against invaders, they really don't kill anything. Their job is to plant the "kiss of death" on an invader – to tag it for destruction. If you go to a fancy wedding, you'll usually pass through a receiving line before you are allowed to enjoy the champagne and cake. Of course, one of the functions of this receiving line is to introduce everyone to the bride and groom. But the other function is to be sure no outsiders are admitted to the celebration. As you pass through the line, you will be screened by someone who is familiar with all the invited guests. If she finds that you don't belong there, she will call the bouncer and have you removed. She doesn't do it herself – certainly not. Her role is to identify undesirables, not to show them to the door. And it's the same with antibodies: they identify invaders, and let other players do the dirty work.

In developed countries, the invaders we encounter most frequently are bacteria and viruses. Antibodies can bind to both types of invaders and tag them for destruction. Immunologists like to say that antibodies can "opsonize" these invaders. This term comes from a German word that means "to prepare for eating." I like to equate opsonize with "decorate," because I picture these bacteria and viruses with antibodies hanging all over them, decorating their surfaces. Anyway, when antibodies opsonize bacteria or viruses, they do so by binding to the invader with their Fab regions, leaving their Fc tails available to bind to Fc receptors on the surface of cells such as macrophages. Using this strategy, antibodies can form a bridge between the invader and the phagocyte (e.g., a macrophage), bringing the invader in close, and preparing it for eating (phagocytosis).

In fact, it's even better than this. When a phagocyte's Fc receptors bind to antibodies that are opsonizing an invader, the appetite of the phagocyte increases, making it even more phagocytic. Macrophages have proteins on their surface that can bind directly to many common invaders. However, the ability of antibodies to form a bridge between a macrophage and an invader allows a macrophage to increase its catalog of enemies to include any invader to which an antibody can bind, common or uncommon. In effect, antibodies focus a macrophage's attention on invaders, some of which (the uncommon ones) a macrophage would otherwise ignore.

During a viral attack, antibodies can do something else that is very important. Viruses enter our cells by binding to certain receptor molecules on a cell's surface. Of course these receptors are not placed there for the convenience of the virus. They are normal receptors, like the Fc receptor, that have quite legitimate functions, but which the virus has learned to use to its own advantage. Once it has bound to these receptors and entered a cell, a virus then uses the cell's machinery to make many copies of itself. These newly made viruses burst out of the cell, sometimes killing it, and go on to infect neighboring cells. Now for the neat part: antibodies can actually bind to a virus while it is still outside of a cell, and can keep the virus either from entering the cell or from replicating once it has entered. Antibodies with these properties are called "neutralizing" antibodies. For example, some neutralizing antibodies can prevent a virus from "docking" on the surface of a cell by binding to the part of the virus that

normally would plug into the cellular receptor. When this happens, the virus is "hung out to dry," opsonized and ready to be eaten by phagocytes!

T cells

Although antibodies can tag viruses for phagocytic ingestion, and can help keep viruses from infecting cells, there is a flaw in the antibody defense against viruses: once a virus gets into a cell, antibodies can't get to it, so the virus is safe to make thousands of copies of itself. Mother Nature recognized this problem, and to deal with it, she invented the famous "killer T cell," another member of the adaptive immune system team.

The importance of T cells is suggested by the fact that an adult human has about 300 billion of them. T cells are very similar to B cells in appearance. In fact, even under an ordinary microscope, an immunologist can't tell them apart. Like B cells, T cells are produced in the bone marrow, and on their surface they display antibody-like molecules called T cell receptors (TCRs). Like the B cell's receptors (the antibody molecules attached to its surface), TCRs also are made by a mix-and-match, modular design strategy. As a result, TCRs are about as diverse as BCRs. T cells also obey the principle of clonal selection: when a T cell's receptors bind to their cognate antigen, the T cell proliferates to build up a clone of T cells with the same specificity. This proliferation stage takes about a week to complete, so like the antibody response, the T cell response is slow and specific.

Although they are similar in many ways, there are also important differences between B cells and T cells. Whereas B cells mature in the bone marrow, T cells mature in the thymus (that's why they're called "T" cells). Further, although B cells make antibodies that can recognize any organic molecule, T cells specialize in recognizing protein antigens. In addition, a B cell can export (secrete) its receptors in the form of antibodies, but a T cell's receptors remain tightly glued to its surface. Perhaps most importantly, a B cell can recognize an antigen "by itself," whereas a T cell, like an old English gentleman, will only recognize an antigen if it is "properly presented" by another cell. I'll explain what this means in a bit.

There are actually three main types of T cells: killer T cells (frequently called cytotoxic lymphocytes – CTLs for short), helper T cells, and regulatory T cells. The killer T cell is a potent weapon that can destroy virus-infected cells. Indeed, by recognizing and killing virus-infected cells, the killer T cell solves the "hiding virus" problem – the flaw I mentioned in the antibody defense against viruses. The way the killer T cell does this is by making contact with its target cell and then triggering it to commit suicide! This "assisted suicide" is a great way to deal with viruses that have infected cells, because when a virus-infected cell dies, the viruses within the cell die also.

The second type of T cell is the helper T cell (Th cell). As you will see, this cell serves as the quarterback of the immune system team. It directs the action by secreting protein molecules called cytokines that have dramatic effects on other immune system cells. These cytokines have names like interleukin 2 (IL-2) and interferon gamma (IFN-γ), and we will discuss what they do in later lectures. For now, it is only important to realize that helper T cells are basically cytokine factories.

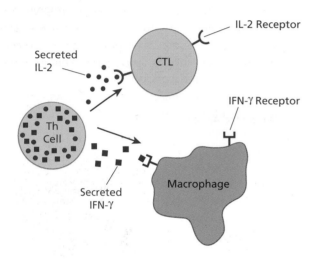

The third type of T cell, the regulatory T cell, is still somewhat mysterious. The role of regulatory T cells is to help keep the immune system from overreacting. However, in some cases, it is not clear how this is accomplished.

Antigen presentation

One thing I need to clear up is exactly how antigen is presented to T cells. It turns out that special proteins called major histocompatibility complex proteins (MHC for short) actually do the "presenting," and that T cells use their receptors to "view" this presented antigen. As you may know, "histo" means tissue, and these major histocompatibility proteins, in addition to being presentation molecules, also are involved in the rejection of transplanted organs. In fact, when you hear that someone is waiting for a "matched" kidney, it's the MHC molecules of the donor and the recipient that the transplant surgeon is trying to match.

There are two types of MHC molecules, called class I and class II. Class I MHC molecules are found in varying amounts on the surface of most cells in the body, and they function as "billboards" that inform killer T cells about what is going on inside these cells. For example, when a human cell is infected by a virus, fragments of viral proteins (called peptides) are loaded onto class I MHC molecules, and transported to the surface of the infected cell. By inspecting these protein fragments displayed by class I MHC molecules, killer T cells can use their receptors to "look into" the cell to determine that it has been infected and that it should be destroyed.

Class II MHC molecules also function as billboards, but this display is intended for the enlightenment of helper T cells. Only certain cells in the body make class II MHC molecules, and these are called antigen presenting cells (APCs for short). Macrophages, for example, are excellent antigen presenting cells. During a bacterial infection, a macrophage will "eat" bacteria, and will load fragments of ingested bacterial proteins onto class II MHC molecules for display on the surface of the macrophage. By using their T cell receptors, helper T cells can scan the macrophage's class II MHC billboards for news of the bacterial infection. So class I MHC molecules alert killer T cells when something isn't right inside a cell, and class II MHC molecules displayed on APCs inform helper T cells that problems exist outside of cells.

Although a class I MHC molecule is made up of one long chain (the heavy chain) plus a short chain (β2-microglobulin), and a class II MHC molecule has two long chains (α and β), you'll notice that these molecules are rather similar in appearance.

Okay, I know it's hard to visualize the real shapes of molecules from drawings like this, so I thought I'd show you a few pictures that may make this more real.

Here's what an empty MHC molecule might look like from the viewpoint of the T cell receptor. Right away you see the groove into which the protein fragment would fit.

Next, let's look at a fully-loaded, class I molecule:

I can tell it's a class I MHC molecule because the peptide is contained nicely within the groove. It turns out that the ends of the groove of a class I molecule are closed, so a protein fragment must be about nine amino acids in length to fit in properly. Class II MHC molecules are slightly different:

Here you see that the peptide overflows the groove. This works fine for class II, because the ends of the groove are open, so protein fragments as large as about 20 amino acids fit nicely.

So MHC molecules resemble buns, and the protein fragments they present resemble wieners. And if you imagine that the cells in our bodies have hot dogs on their surfaces, you won't be far wrong about antigen presentation. That's certainly the way I picture it!

Activation of the adaptive immune system

Because B and T cells are such potent weapons, Mother Nature put into place the requirement that cells of the adaptive immune system must be activated before they can function. Collectively, B and T cells are called lymphocytes, and how they are activated is one of the key issues in immunology. To introduce this concept, I will sketch how helper T cells are activated.

The first step in the activation of a helper T cell is recognition of its cognate antigen (e.g., a fragment of a bacterial protein) displayed by class II MHC molecules on the surface of an antigen presenting cell. But seeing its cognate antigen on that billboard isn't enough – a second signal or "key" is also required for activation. This second signal is non-specific (it's the same for any antigen), and it involves a protein (B7 in this drawing) on the surface of an antigen presenting cell that plugs into its receptor (CD28 in this drawing) on the surface of the helper T cell.

You see an example of this kind of two-key system when you visit your safe deposit box. You bring with you a key that is specific for your box – it won't fit any other. The bank teller provides a second, non-specific key that will fit all the boxes. Only when both keys are inserted into the locks on your box can it be opened. Your specific key alone won't do it, and the teller's non-specific key alone won't either. You need both. Now, why do you suppose helper T cells and other cells of the adaptive immune system require two keys for activation? For safety, of course – just like your bank box. These cells are powerful weapons that must only be activated at the appropriate time and place.

Once a helper T cell has been activated by this two-key system, it proliferates to build up a clone composed of many helper T cells whose receptors recognize the same antigen. These helper cells then mature into cells that can produce the cytokines needed to direct the activities of the immune system. B cells and killer T cells also require two-key systems for their activation, and we'll talk about them in another lecture.

The secondary lymphoid organs

If you've been thinking about how the adaptive immune system might get turned on during an attack, you've probably begun to wonder whether this could ever happen. After all, there are probably only about 10 000 T cells that will have TCRs specific for a given invader, and for these T cells to be activated, they must come in contact with an antigen presenting cell that also has "seen" the invader. Given that these T cells and APCs are spread all over the body, it would not seem very likely that this would happen before an invasion got completely out of hand. Fortunately, to make this system work with reasonable probability, Mother Nature invented the "secondary lymphoid organs," the best known of which is the lymph node. You may not be familiar with the lymphatic system, so I'd better say a few words about it.

In your home, you have two plumbing systems. The first supplies the water that comes out of your faucets. This is a pressurized system, with the pressure being provided by a pump. In addition, you also have another plumbing system that includes the drains in your sinks, showers, and toilets. This second system is not under pressure – the water just flows down the drain and out into the sewer. The two systems are connected in the sense that eventually the waste-water is recycled and used again.

The plumbing in a human is very much like this. We have a pressurized system (the cardiovascular system) in which blood is pumped around the body by the heart. Everybody knows about this one. But we also have another plumbing system: the lymphatic system. This system is not under pressure, and it drains the fluid (lymph) that leaks out of our blood vessels into our tissues. Without this system, our tissues would fill up with fluid and we'd look like the Pillsbury Doughboy. Fortunately, lymph is collected from the tissues of our lower body into lymphatic vessels, and is transported by these vessels, under the influence of muscular contraction, through a series of one-way valves to the upper torso. This lymph, plus lymph from the left side of the upper torso, is collected into the thoracic duct and emptied into the left subclavian vein to be recycled back into the blood. Likewise, lymph from the right side of the upper

body is collected into the right lymphatic duct and is emptied into the right subclavian vein. From this diagram, you can see that as the lymph winds its way back to be reunited with the blood, it passes through a series of way stations – the lymph nodes.

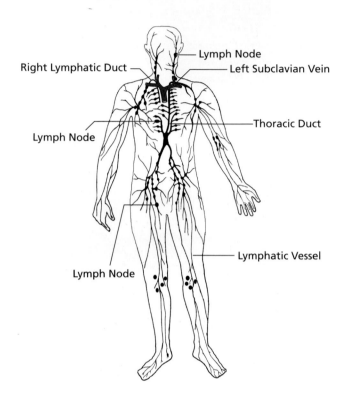

There are thousands of lymph nodes that range in size from very small to almost as big as a Brussels sprout. Invaders like bacteria and viruses are carried by the lymph to nearby nodes, and antigen presenting cells that have picked up foreign antigens in the tissues travel to lymph nodes to present their cargo. Meanwhile, B cells and T cells circulate from node to node, looking for the antigens for which they are "fated." So lymph nodes really function as "dating bars" – places where T cells, B cells, APCs, and antigen all gather for the purposes of communication and activation. By bringing these cells and antigens together within the small volume of a lymph node, Mother Nature increases the probability that they will interact to efficiently activate the adaptive immune system.

Immunological memory

After B and T cells have been activated, have proliferated to build up clones of cells with identical antigen specificities, and have vanquished the enemy, most of them die off. This is a good idea, because we wouldn't want our immune systems to fill up with old B and T cells. On the other hand, it would be nice if some of these experienced B and T cells would stick around, just in case we are exposed to the same invaders again. That way, the adaptive immune system wouldn't have to start from scratch. And that's just the way it works. These "leftover" B and T cells are called memory cells, and in addition to being more numerous than the original, inexperienced B and T cells, memory cells are easier to activate. As a result of this immunological memory, the adaptive system usually can spring into action so quickly during a second attack that you never even experience any symptoms.

Tolerance of self

As I mentioned earlier, B cell receptors and T cell receptors are so diverse that they should be able to recognize any potential invader. This raises a problem, however, because if the receptors are this diverse, many of them are certain to recognize our own "self" molecules (e.g., the molecules that make up our cells, or proteins like insulin that circulate in our blood). If this were to happen, our adaptive immune system might attack our own bodies, and we could die from autoimmune disease. Fortunately, Mother Nature has devised ways to educate B cells and T cells to discriminate between ourselves and dangerous invaders. Although the mechanisms involved in teaching B and T cells to be tolerant of our self antigens still are not completely understood, the education which B and T cells receive is sufficiently rigorous that autoimmune disease is relatively rare.

A COMPARISON OF THE INNATE AND ADAPTIVE IMMUNE SYSTEMS

Now that you have met some of the main players, I want to emphasize the differences between the innate and adaptive immune system "teams." Understanding how they differ is crucial to understanding how the immune system works.

Imagine that you are in the middle of town and someone steals your shoes. You look around for a store where you can buy another pair, and the first store you see is called Charlie's Custom Shoes. This store has shoes of every style, color, and size, and the salesperson is able to fit you in exactly the shoes you need. However, when it comes time to pay, you are told that you must wait a week or two to get your shoes – they will have to be custom-made for you, and that will take a while. But you need shoes right now! You are barefoot, and you must have something to put on your feet until those custom shoes arrive. So they send you across the street to Freddie's Fast Fit – a store that only carries a few styles and sizes. Freddie's wouldn't be able to fit Shaquille O'Neal, but this store does stock shoes in the common sizes that fit most people – so you can get a pair right away to tide you over until your custom shoes are made for you.

This is very similar to the way the innate and adaptive immune systems work. The players of the innate system (like the macrophage) are already in place, and are ready to defend against relatively small quantities of the invaders we are likely to meet on a day-to-day basis. In many instances, the innate system is so effective and so fast that the adaptive immune system never even kicks in. In other cases, the innate system may be insufficient to deal with the invasion, and the adaptive system will need to be mobilized. This takes a while, however, because the B and T cells of the adaptive system must be custom-made through the process of clonal selection and proliferation. Meanwhile, the innate immune system must do its best to hold the invaders at bay.

THE INNATE SYSTEM RULES!

Until fairly recently, immunologists thought that the only function of the innate system was to provide a rapid defense which would deal with invaders while the adaptive immune system was getting cranked up. However, it is now clear that the innate system does much more than that.

The adaptive immune system's antigen receptors (BCRs and TCRs) are so diverse that they can probably recognize any protein molecule in the universe. However, the adaptive system is clueless as to which of these molecules is dangerous and which is not. So how does the adaptive system distinguish friend from foe? The answer is that it relies on the judgment of the innate system.

In contrast to the antigen receptors of the adaptive immune system, which are totally "unfocused," the receptors of the innate system are precisely tuned to detect the presence of the common pathogens (disease-causing agents) we encounter in daily life – viruses, bacteria, fungi, and parasites. In addition, the innate system has receptors that can detect when "uncommon" pathogens kill human cells. Consequently, it is the innate system which is responsible for sensing danger and for activating the adaptive immune system. In a real sense, the innate system gives "permission" to the adaptive system to respond to an invasion. But it's even better than that, because the innate system does more than just turn the adaptive system on. The innate system actually integrates all the information it collects about an invader, and formulates a plan of action. This "game plan," which the innate system delivers to the adaptive immune system, tells which weapons to mobilize (e.g., B cells or killer T cells) and exactly where in the body these weapons should be deployed. So if we think of the helper T cell as the quarterback of the adaptive immune system team, we should consider the innate immune system to be the "coach" – for it is the innate system which "scouts" the opponents, designs the game plan, and sends in the plays for the quarterback to call.

EPILOGUE

We have come to the end of our turbo overview of the immune system, and by now you should have a rough idea of how the system works. In the next nine lectures, we will focus more sharply on the individual players of the innate and adaptive system teams, paying special attention to how and where these players interact with each other to make the system function efficiently.

LECTURE 2

The Innate Immune System

For years, immunologists didn't pay much attention to the innate system – perhaps because the adaptive system seemed more interesting. However, studies of the adaptive immune system have led to a new appreciation of the role that the innate system plays, not only as a lightning-fast, second line of defense (if we count physical barriers as our first defense), but also as an activator and a controller of the adaptive immune system.

It's easy to understand the importance of the innate system's quick response to common invaders if you think about what could happen in an uncontrolled bacterial infection. Imagine that the splinter from your hot tub deck introduced just one bacterium into your tissues. As you know, bacteria multiply very quickly. In fact, a single bacterium doubling in number every 30 minutes could give rise to roughly 100 trillion bacteria in one day. If you've ever worked with bacterial cultures, you know that a one liter culture containing one trillion bacteria is so dense you can't see through it. So, a single bacterium proliferating for one day could yield a dense culture of about 100 liters. Now remember that your total blood volume is only about five liters, and you can appreciate what an unchecked bacterial infection could do to a human! Without the quick-acting innate immune system to defend us, we would clearly be in big trouble.

The weapons of the innate immune system include the complement proteins, the professional phagocytes, and natural killer cells. We'll begin our discussion with my favorite:

THE COMPLEMENT SYSTEM

The complement system is composed of about 20 different proteins that work together to destroy invaders and to signal other immune system players that the attack is on. The complement system is very old. Even sea urchins, which evolved about 700 million years ago, have a complement system. In humans, complement proteins begin to be made during the first trimester of fetal development, so it's clear that Mother Nature wants this important system to be ready to go, well before a child is born. Indeed, those rare humans born with a defect in one of the major complement proteins usually do not live long before succumbing to infection.

When I first read about the complement system, I thought it was way too complicated to even bother understanding. But as I studied it further, I began to realize that it is really quite simple and elegant. As with just about everything else in the immune defense, the complement system must be activated before it can function, and there are three ways this can happen. The first, the so-called "classical" pathway, depends on antibodies for activation, so we'll save that for a later lecture. Because the way the complement system functions is independent of how it is activated, you won't miss much by waiting until later to hear about the antibody-dependent pathway of activation.

The alternative pathway

The second way the complement system can be activated is called the "alternative" pathway – although in evolutionary terms, the alternative pathway certainly evolved before the classical pathway. Immunologists call the antibody-dependent activation "classical," simply because it happened to be discovered first.

The proteins that make up the complement system are produced mainly by the liver, and are present at high concentrations in blood and tissues. The most abundant complement protein is called C3, and in the human body, C3 molecules are continually being broken into two smaller proteins. One of the protein fragments created by this "spontaneous" cleavage, C3b, is very reactive, and can bind to either of two common, chemical groups (amino or hydroxyl groups). Because many of the proteins and carbohydrates that make up the surfaces of invaders (e.g., bacterial cells) have amino or hydroxyl groups, there are lots of targets for these little C3b "grenades."

Surface of Bacterium

If C3b doesn't find one of these chemical groups to react with within about 60 microseconds, it is neutralized by binding to a water molecule, and the game is over. So the spontaneously clipped C3 molecule has to be right up close to the surface of a cell in order for the complement cascade to continue. Once C3b is stabilized by reacting with a molecule on the surface of an invader, another complement protein, B, binds to C3b, and complement protein D comes along and clips off part of B to yield C3bBb.

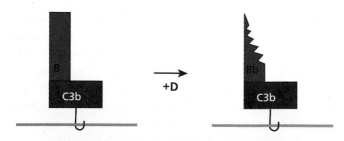

Once a bacterium has this C3bBb molecule glued to its surface, the fun really begins, because C3bBb acts like a "chain saw" that can cut other C3 proteins and convert them to C3b. Consequently, C3 molecules that are in the neighborhood don't have to wait for spontaneous clipping events to convert them to C3b – the C3bBb molecule (called a convertase) can do the job very efficiently. And once another C3 molecule has been clipped, it too can bind to an amino or hydroxyl group on the surface of the bacterium.

This process can continue, and pretty soon there will be lots of C3b molecules attached to the surface of the target bacterium – and each of them can form a C3bBb convertase which can then cut even more C3 molecules. All this attaching and cutting sets up a positive feedback loop, and the whole process just snowballs:

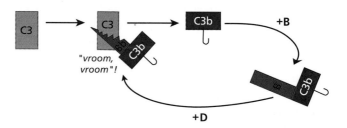

"vroom, vroom"!

Once C3b is bound to the surface of a bacterium, the complement cascade can proceed further. The C3bBb chain saw can cut off part of another complement protein, C5, and the clipped product, C5b, can combine with other complement proteins (C6, C7, C8, and C9) to make a "membrane attack complex" (MAC for short). To form this structure, C5b, C6, C7, and C8 form a "stalk" that anchors the complex in the bacterial cell wall. Then C9 proteins are added to make a channel that opens up a hole in the surface of the bacterium. And once a bacterium has a hole in its surface, it's toast!

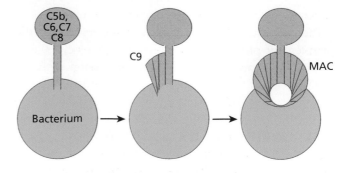

I have used a bacterium as our "model pathogen," but the complement system also can defend against other invaders such as parasites and even some viruses. Now, you may be wondering: with these grenades going off all over the place, why doesn't the complement system form membrane attack complexes on the surface of our own cells? The answer is that human cells are equipped with many safeguards that keep this from happening. In fact, Mother Nature was so worried about the complement system reacting inappropriately that she devoted about as many proteins to controlling the complement system as there are proteins in the system itself. For instance, the complement fragment, C3b, can be clipped to an inactive form by proteins in the blood, and this clipping is accelerated by an enzyme (MCP) that is present on the surface of human cells. There is also a protein on human cells called decay accelerating factor (DAF) which accelerates the destruction of the convertase, C3bBb, by other blood proteins. This can keep the positive feedback loop from getting started. And yet another cell-surface protein, CD59 (also called protectin), can kick almost-finished MACs off before they can make a hole in one of our cells.

There's an interesting story that illustrates why these safeguards are so important. As you know, transplant surgeons don't have enough human organs to satisfy the demand for transplantation, so they are considering using organs from animals. One of the hot candidates for an organ donor is the pig, because pigs are cheap to raise, and their organs are about the same size as those of humans. As a warm-up for human transplantation, surgeons decided to transplant a pig organ into a baboon. This experiment was not a big success. Almost immediately, the baboon's immune system began to attack the organ, and within minutes the transplanted organ was a bloody pulp. The culprit? The complement system. It turns out that the pig versions of DAF and CD59 don't work to control primate complement, so the unprotected pig organ was vulnerable to attack by the baboon's complement system.

This story highlights two important features of the complement system. First, **the complement system works very fast.** These complement proteins are present at high concentrations in blood and in tissues, and they are ready to go against any invader that has a surface with a spare hydroxyl or amino group. A second characteristic of this system is that **if a cell surface is not protected, it will be attacked by complement. In fact, the picture you should have is that the complement system is continually dropping these little grenades, and any unprotected surface will be a target. In this system, the default option is death!**

The lectin activation pathway

In addition to the classical (antibody-dependent) and alternative (antibody-independent) pathways of complement activation, there is a third pathway that may be the most important activation pathway of all. The central player in this pathway is a protein that is produced mainly in the liver, and which is present in moderate concentrations in the blood and tissues. This protein is called mannose-binding lectin (MBL for short). A lectin is a protein that is able to bind to a carbohydrate molecule, and mannose is a carbohydrate molecule found on the surface of many common pathogens. For example, mannose-binding lectin has been shown to bind to yeasts such as *Candida albicans*; to viruses such as HIV-1 and influenza A; to many bacteria including *Salmonella* and *Streptococcus*; and to parasites like *Leishmania*. In contrast, mannose-binding lectin does not bind to the carbohydrates found on healthy human cells and tissues. This is an example of an important strategy employed by the innate system: **the innate system mainly focuses on patterns of carbohydrates and fats that are found on the surfaces of common pathogens.**

The way mannose-binding lectin works to activate the complement system is very simple. In the blood, MBL binds to another protein called MASP. Then, when the mannose-binding lectin grabs its target (mannose on the surface of a bacterium, for example), the MASP protein functions like a convertase to clip C3 complement proteins to make C3b. Because C3 is so abundant in the blood, this happens very efficiently. The C3b fragments can then bind to the surface of the bacterium, and the complement chain reaction we just discussed will be off and running. So, **whereas the alternative activation pathway is spontaneous, and can be visualized as "grenades" going off randomly here and there to destroy any unprotected surface, lectin activation can be thought of as "smart bombs" that are targeted by mannose-binding lectins.**

Other functions of the complement system

In addition to building membrane attack complexes, the complement system has two other functions in innate immunity. When C3b has attached itself to the surface of an invader, it can be clipped by a serum protein to produce a smaller fragment, iC3b. The "i" prefix denotes that this cleaved protein is now inactive for making MACs. However, it is still glued to the invader, and it can prepare the invader for phagocytosis (i.e., can opsonize it) in much the same way that invaders can be opsonized by antibodies. On the surface of phagocytes (e.g., macrophages) are receptors that can bind to iC3b, and the binding of iC3b-opsonized invaders facilitates phagocytosis. Many invaders have surfaces that are rather "slimy," making them difficult for macrophages to grasp. However, when these slippery invaders are coated with complement fragments, phagocytes can get a better grip. Thus, **a second function of complement is to decorate the surfaces of invaders, thereby acting like a poor man's antibody in opsonization.**

The complement system has a third important function: **fragments of complement proteins can serve as chemoattractants – chemicals that recruit other immune system players to the battle site.** For example, C3a and C5a are the pieces of C3 and C5 that are clipped off when C3b and C5b are made (let nothing be wasted!). These fragments don't bind to the surface of invaders. Rather, they are set free in the tissues, where they attract macrophages and neutrophils, and activate these cells so that they become more potent killers. Interestingly, these fragments, C3a and C5a, are called anaphylatoxins, because they can contribute to anaphylactic shock – something we will talk about in another lecture.

So the complement system is quite multifunctional. **It can destroy invaders by building membrane attack complexes. It can enhance the function of phagocytic cells by tickling their complement receptors. And it can alert other cells that we are being attacked. Most importantly, it can do all these things very fast.**

PROFESSIONAL PHAGOCYTES

Professional phagocytes comprise the second arm of the innate system. These cells are called "professional" because they make their living mainly by eating (phagocytosis). The most important of the professional phagocytes are the macrophages and the neutrophils.

Macrophages – the immune system's sentinels

Macrophages are found under your skin, where they provide protection against invaders which penetrate this barrier and gain entry into your tissues (e.g., as the result of a wound or a burn). Macrophages also are present in your lungs, where they defend against inhaled microbes. Still other macrophages reside in the tissues that surround your intestines. There they lie in wait for microbial invaders you have ingested, and which have escaped the confines of your intestines and have entered your tissues. Indeed, macrophages are sentinel cells which can be found just below the surface of all areas of your body which are exposed to the outside world – areas that are prime targets for microbial infection.

Macrophages can exist in three stages of readiness. In tissues, macrophages are usually found just lounging and slowly proliferating. In this "resting" state, they function primarily as garbage collectors, taking sips of whatever is around them, and keeping our tissues free of debris. About one million cells die per second in an adult human, so macrophages have a lot of tidying up to do! Dying cells give off "find me" signals that attract macrophages, and bring them close enough to recognize "eat me" signals displayed on the surface of dying cells.

While resting, macrophages express very few class II MHC molecules on their surfaces, so they aren't much good at presenting antigen to helper T cells. This makes sense. Why would they want to present garbage anyway? For the average macrophage, life is pretty boring. They live for months in tissues and just collect garbage.

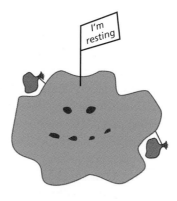

Every once in a while, however, some of these resting macrophages receive signals which alert them that the barrier defense has been penetrated, and that there are intruders in the area. When this happens, they become activated (or "primed," as immunologists usually say). In this state, macrophages take larger gulps and upregulate expression of class II MHC molecules. Now a macrophage can function as an antigen presenting cell, and when it engulfs invaders, it can use its class II MHC molecules to display fragments of the invaders' proteins for helper T cells to see. Although a number of different signals can prime a resting macrophage, the best studied is an intercellular communication molecule (cytokine) called interferon gamma (IFN-γ). This cytokine is produced mainly by helper T cells and natural killer cells.

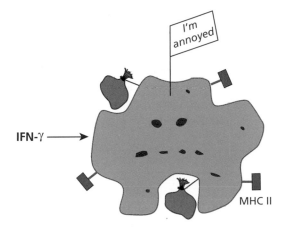

IFN-γ Receptor

In the primed state, macrophages are good antigen presenters and reasonably good killers. However, there is an even higher state of readiness, "hyperactivation," which they can attain if they receive a direct signal from an invader. For example, such a signal can be conveyed by a molecule called lipopolysaccharide (LPS for short). LPS, a component of the outer cell wall of Gram-negative bacteria like *Escherichia coli*, can be shed by these bacteria, and can bind to receptors on the surface of primed macrophages. Macrophages also have receptors for mannose – the carbohydrate that is an ingredient of the cell walls of many common pathogens and which, as we discussed earlier, is a "danger signal" that can activate the complement system. When receptors on the surface of the macrophage bind to either LPS or mannose, the macrophage knows for sure that there has been an invasion. Faced with this realization, the macrophage stops proliferating, and focuses its attention on killing. In the hyperactive state, macrophages grow larger and increase their rate of phagocytosis. In fact, they become so large and phagocytic that they can ingest invaders that are as big as unicellular parasites. Hyperactivated macrophages also produce and secrete another cytokine, tumor necrosis factor (TNF). This cytokine can kill tumor cells and virus-infected cells, and can help activate other immune system warriors.

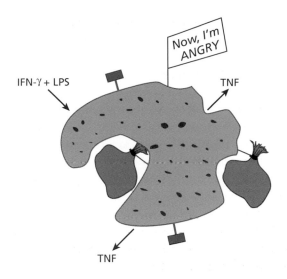

Inside a hyperactivated macrophage, the number of lysosomes increases, so that the destruction of ingested invaders becomes more efficient. In addition, hyperactivated macrophages increase production of reactive oxygen molecules like hydrogen peroxide. You know what peroxide can do to hair, so you can imagine what it might do to a bacterium! Finally, when hyperactivated, a macrophage can dump the contents of its lysosomes onto multicellular parasites, enabling it to destroy invaders that are too large to "eat." Yes, a hyperactivated macrophage is a killing machine!

So **a macrophage is a very versatile cell. It can function as a garbage collector, as an antigen presenting cell, or as a vicious killer – depending on its activation level.** However, you shouldn't get the impression that macrophages have three "gears." Nothing in immunology has gears, and the activation state of a macrophage is a continuum that really depends both on the type and the strength of the activation signals it receives.

Usually, macrophages are able to deal with small attacks. However, when invaders are numerous, macrophages risk being overpowered, and in these cases, macrophages call for backup. The most common reinforcement for battling macrophages is another cell called a neutrophil. Indeed, **although the macrophage is unmatched in versatility, the most important of the professional phagocytes is probably the neutrophil.**

Neutrophils – the immune system's foot soldiers

All of our cells receive their nutrients from the blood, and consequently, no cell is more than about the thickness of a fingernail from a blood vessel. If a cell is farther away than that, it will die of starvation. Because our tissues are laced with blood vessels, blood is the perfect vehicle for bringing reinforcements to those parts of the body which are under attack, and circulating through our veins and arteries are about 20 billion neutrophils. In contrast to macrophages, which can be thought of as sentinels, neutrophils are more like "foot soldiers." Their job is to "kill things and break stuff" – and like our armed forces, they are really good at this.

Neutrophils live a very short time. In fact, they come out of the bone marrow programmed to die in an average of about five days. Interestingly, they die by committing suicide, a process known as "apoptosis." In contrast to macrophages, neutrophils are not antigen presenting cells. They are professional killers which are "on call" from the blood.

Once they have been summoned, it only takes neutrophils about half an hour to exit the blood and become fully activated. In this state, neutrophils are incredibly phagocytic, and once their prey has been taken inside, a whole battery of powerful chemicals awaits the unlucky "guest." Neutrophils also produce battle cytokines (e.g., TNF) that can alert other immune system cells. And most importantly, activated neutrophils give off destructive chemicals which are pre-made and stored inside the neutrophil until needed. These chemicals can turn tissues into a "toxic soup" that is lethal to invading microbes. Indeed, neutrophils are unique in that they are the only immune system cells that are "licensed" to liquify both cells and connective tissue.

My friend, Dan Tenen, studies neutrophils. Another friend, Linda Clayton, who experiments with T cells, likes to kid him by asking, "Why do you bother studying neutrophils, Dan? All they do is dive into pus and die!" She's right, of course. Pus is mainly dead neutrophils. However, Dan reminds her that humans can live for long periods without her fancy T cells, but without his neutrophils, they will succumb to infection and die within a matter of days.

Now, why do you think Mother Nature set things up so that macrophages are very long lived, yet neutrophils live only a few days? Doesn't that seem wasteful? Why not let neutrophils enjoy a long life, just like macrophages? That's right! It would be too dangerous. Neutrophils come out of blood vessels ready to kill, and in the course of this killing, there is always damage to normal tissues. So to limit that damage, neutrophils are programmed to be short-lived. If the battle requires additional neutrophils, more can be recruited from the blood – there are plenty of them there. In contrast, macrophages

act as sentinels that watch for invaders and signal the attack. Consequently, it makes sense that macrophages should live a long time out in the tissues.

How neutrophils exit the blood stream

You may be wondering: If neutrophils are all that dangerous, how do they know when to leave the blood stream and where to go? It certainly wouldn't do to have neutrophils leave the blood and become activated just any old place. No indeed, and the way this works is very clever. Inside blood vessels, neutrophils exist in an inactive state, and they are swept along by the blood at a high rate of speed: about 1000 microns per second. If you're the size of a neutrophil, that's really fast.

NORMAL TISSUE

In this sketch, you will notice that there is a protein, ICAM (short for intercellular adhesion molecule), which is expressed on the surface of the endothelial cells that line blood vessels. There is also another adhesion molecule called selectin ligand (SLIG) that is expressed on the surface of neutrophils. As you can see, however, these two adhesion molecules are not "partners," so they don't bind to each other, and the neutrophil is free to zip along with the flowing blood.

Now imagine that you get a splinter in your big toe, and that the bacteria on the splinter activate macrophages which are standing guard in the tissues of your foot. These activated macrophages give off cytokines, interleukin 1 (IL-1) and TNF, which signal that an invasion has begun. When endothelial cells that line nearby blood vessels receive these alarm signals, they begin to express a new protein on their surface called selectin (SEL). It normally takes about six hours for this protein to be made and transported to the surface of endothelial cells. Selectin is the adhesion partner for selectin ligand, so when selectin is expressed on the endothelial cell surface, it functions like Velcro to grab neutrophils as they fly by. However, this interaction between selectin and its ligand is only strong enough to cause neutrophils to slow down and roll along the inner surface of the blood vessel.

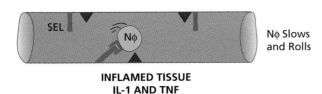

**INFLAMED TISSUE
IL-1 AND TNF**

As a neutrophil rolls, it "sniffs." What it's sniffing for is a signal that there is a battle (an inflammatory reaction) going on in the tissues. The complement fragment, C5a, and the bacterial wall component, LPS, are two of the inflammatory signals that a neutrophil recognizes. When it receives such signals, the neutrophil rushes a new protein called integrin (INT) to its surface. This quick reaction is important, because the neutrophil hasn't stopped – it's still rolling along. If it rolls too far, it will leave the region where selectin is expressed, and the neutrophil will start to zoom along again at "blood speed." To make rapid surface expression of integrin possible, a lot of this protein is made in advance by the neutrophil, and is stored inside the cell until needed.

When integrin appears on the neutrophil's surface, it interacts with its binding partner, ICAM, which is expressed on the surface of endothelial cells. This interaction is very strong, and it causes the neutrophil to stop rolling.

**INFLAMED TISSUE
C5a AND LPS**

Once a neutrophil has stopped, it can be influenced by molecules called chemoattractants to pry apart the endothelial cells that line the blood vessels, exit into the tissues, and migrate to the site of inflammation. These chemoattractants include C5a, as well as fragments of bacterial proteins called f-met peptides.

**FOLLOWS "SCENT" OF
f-met AND C5a**

All bacterial proteins begin with a special initiator amino acid called formyl methionine (f-met). Less than 0.1% of all human proteins contain this amino acid, so f-met peptides are relatively unique to bacteria. As they ingest bacteria, macrophages burp up f-met peptides, and neutrophils that have exited the blood can follow the trail of these f-met peptides to find the battle. In addition, cytokines such as TNF activate neutrophils as they travel through the tissues, so they arrive at the battle scene ready to kill.

Neutrophil logic

This system – which involves selectin–selectin ligand binding to make the neutrophil roll, integrin–ICAM interactions to stop the neutrophil, and chemoattractants and their receptors on the neutrophil to facilitate exit from the blood – may seem a little over complicated. Wouldn't it be simpler just to have one pair of adhesion molecules (say, selectin and its ligand) do all three things? Yes, it would be simpler, but it would also be very dangerous. In a human there are about 100 billion endothelial cells. Suppose one of them gets a little crazy, and begins to express a lot of selectin on its surface. If selectin binding were the only requirement, neutrophils could empty out of the blood into normal tissues where they could do terrible damage. Having three types of molecules which must be expressed before neutrophils can exit the blood and spring into action helps make the system failsafe.

You remember I mentioned that to completely upregulate expression of that first cellular adhesion molecule, selectin, takes about six hours. Doesn't this seem a bit too leisurely? Wouldn't it be better to begin recruiting neutrophils from the blood just as soon as a macrophage senses danger? Not really. Before you start to recruit reinforcements, you want to be sure that the attack is serious. If a macrophage encounters only a few invaders, it can usually handle the situation without help in a short time. In contrast, a major invasion involving many macrophages can go on for days. The sustained expression of alarm cytokines from many macrophages engaged in battle is required to upregulate selectin expression, and this insures that more troops will be summoned only when they really are needed.

Neutrophils are not the only blood cells that need to exit the blood and enter tissues. For example, eosinophils and mast cells, which are involved in protection against parasites, must exit the blood at the site of a parasitic infection. Monocytes, which can mature into tissue macrophages, also need to leave the blood stream at appropriate places. In addition, B cells and T cells must exit the blood and enter lymph nodes, where they can be activated. And once they are activated, these cells must then be dispatched to sites of infection. This whole business is like a mail system in which there are trillions of packages (immune system cells) that must be delivered to the correct destinations. This delivery problem is solved by using the same basic strategy that works so well for neutrophils. The key feature of the immune system's "postal service" is that the Velcro-like molecules which cause the cells to roll and stop are different from cell type to cell type and destination to destination. As a result, these cellular adhesion molecules actually serve as "zip codes" to insure that cells are delivered to the appropriate locations. Indeed, the selectins and their ligands are really families of molecules, and only certain members of the selectin family will pair up with certain members of the selectin ligand family. The same is true of the integrins and their ligands. Because of this two-digit zip code (type of selectin, type of integrin), there are enough "addresses" available to send the many different immune system cells to all the right places. **By equipping immune system cells with different adhesion molecules, and by equipping their intended destinations with the corresponding adhesion partners, Mother Nature makes sure that the different types of immune system cells will roll, stop, and exit the blood exactly where they are needed.**

NATURAL KILLER CELLS

In addition to the complement system and the professional phagocytes, there is a third important player on the innate immune system team – the natural killer (NK) cell. Natural killer cells are descended from blood stem cells, as are all the rest of the blood cells, and although natural killer cells are members of the "lymphocyte" family – together with B cells and T cells – NK cells do not have receptors which are made by mixing and matching gene segments. Natural killer cells mature in the bone marrow as do B cells, but NK cells are short lived, with a half-life of only about a week.

NK cells are not sentinel cells like macrophages, which hang out in our tissues and wait for invaders. Indeed, very few NK cells are found in tissues that are not under attack. Like neutrophils, NK cells are "on call," and most NK cells are found in the blood or in the spleen and liver (two organs that store blood). Natural killer cells use the "roll, stop, exit" strategy to leave the blood and enter tissues at sites of infection, and once in the tissues, NK cells proliferate rapidly to build up their numbers. When they reach the battleground, natural killer cells can play

two roles in defending us against infections. First, **when NK cells receive battle signals from other immune system cells, they can give off cytokines that help with the defense.**

In addition to functioning as cytokine factories, **natural killer cells can destroy tumor cells, virus-infected cells, bacteria, parasites, and fungi. NK cells kill these cells by forcing them to commit suicide.** In some cases, NK cells employ an "injection system" that uses perforin proteins to deliver "suicide" enzymes (e.g., granzyme B) into a target cell. In other situations, a protein called Fas ligand on the NK cell surface interacts with a protein called Fas on the surface of its target, signaling the target cell to self-destruct.

The method NK cells employ to identify their targets is quite different from that of killer T cells. Natural killer cells have no T cell receptors, but they have two other types of receptors on their surface: "activating" receptors which, when engaged, motivate the NK cell to kill; and "inhibitory" receptors which, when engaged, encourage it not to kill.

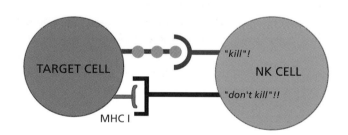

The "don't kill" signal is conveyed by receptors that recognize class I MHC molecules on the surface of a potential target cell. Class I MHC molecules are found in varying amounts on the surface of most healthy cells in our bodies. Consequently, the presence of this surface molecule is an indication that a cell is doing okay. In contrast, the "kill" signals involve interactions between the activating receptors on the surface of an NK cell and unusual carbohydrates or proteins on the surface of a target cell. These peculiar surface molecules act as flags which indicate that the target cell has been "stressed," usually because it has been infected with a virus or is becoming cancerous. **It is the balance between the "kill" and the "don't kill" signals which determines whether NK cells will destroy a target cell.**

Now, why do you think it would be a good idea to have NK cells destroy target cells that do not express class I MHC molecules? You remember that by examining peptides displayed by class I MHC proteins, killer T cells are able to "look inside" cells to see if anything is wrong. But what if some clever virus were to turn off expression of MHC molecules in the cells it infects? Wouldn't those virus-infected cells then be "invisible" to killer T cells? Indeed they would be. So, in those cases, it would be great to have another weapon that could kill virus-infected cells that don't display MHC molecules on their surface. And that's just what natural killer cells can do.

Like macrophages, NK cells contain granules which enclose destructive enzymes and chemicals, and like macrophages, NK cells can exist in several stages of readiness. Resting NK cells produce some cytokines and can kill, but they produce larger quantities of cytokines and can kill better if they are activated. **Several signals have been identified that can activate natural killer cells, and each of these signals is generated only when the body is under attack.** For example, NK cells can be activated when their surface receptors detect the bacterial cell wall component, LPS. NK cells can also be activated by warning proteins called interferon alpha (IFN-α) and interferon beta (IFN-β), which usually are given off by cells when they are being attacked by viruses.

So **natural killer cells are rather like killer T cells and helper T cells all rolled into one. NK cells can destroy infected cells, just as killer T cells can. In addition, like helper T cells, NK cells can function as cytokine factories.**

THE INNATE IMMUNE SYSTEM – A COOPERATIVE EFFORT

To make the innate system work efficiently, there must be cooperation between players on the innate team. For example, neutrophils are "on call" from the blood. And who does the calling? The sentinel cell, the macrophage. So here we have a defense strategy in which "garbage collectors" alert the "hired guns" when their help is needed. Indeed, cooperation between macrophages and neutrophils is essential for mounting an effective defense against invading microbes. Without macrophages to summon them to sites of attack, neutrophils would just go around and around in the blood. And without neutrophils, macrophages would be hard pressed to deal with sizable infections.

Also, during a bacterial infection, molecules like LPS bind to receptors on the surface of natural killer cells, signaling that an attack is on. NK cells then respond by producing significant amounts of IFN-γ.

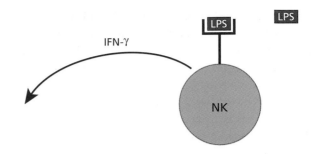

The IFN-γ produced by NK cells can prime macrophages, which can then be hyperactivated when their receptors also bind to LPS.

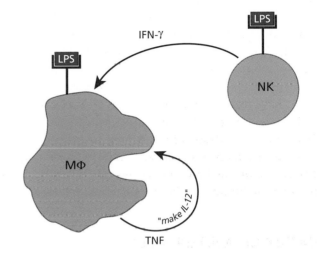

When a macrophage is hyperactivated, it produces lots of TNF. A macrophage also has receptors on its surface to which this cytokine can bind, and when TNF binds to these receptors, the macrophage begins to secrete IL-12. Together, TNF and IL-12 influence NK cells to increase the amount of IFN-γ they produce. And when there is more IFN-γ around, more macrophages can be primed.

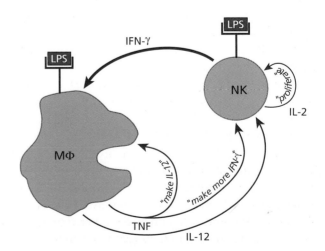

There is something else interesting going on here. IL-2 is a growth factor that is produced by NK cells. Normally, NK cells don't express the receptor for IL-2, so they don't proliferate in response to this cytokine – even though they are making it. During an infection, however, macrophages produce TNF, which upregulates the expression of IL-2 receptors on the surface of NK cells. Consequently, NK cells can now react to the IL-2 they make and begin to proliferate. As a result of this proliferation, there will soon be many more NK cells to defend against an invasion – and to help activate more macrophages. So macrophages and NK cells cooperate in several different ways to strengthen the response of the innate system to an attack.

Professional phagocytes and the complement system also work together. As we discussed, complement protein fragments such as iC3b can tag invaders for phagocyte ingestion. But complement opsonization also can play a role in activating macrophages. When C3 fragments that are decorating an invader bind to receptors on the surface of a macrophage, this provides an activation signal for the macrophage which is similar to that supplied by LPS. This is a good idea, because there are invaders that can be opsonized by complement, but which do not make LPS.

Cooperation between the complement system and the phagocytes is not a one-way street. Activated macrophages actually produce several of the most important complement proteins: C3, factor B, and factor D. So in the heat of battle, when complement proteins may be depleted out in the tissues, macrophages can help resupply the complement system. In addition, during an infection, macrophages secrete chemicals that increase the permeability of nearby blood vessels. And when these vessels become leaky, more complement proteins are released into the tissues.

All these interactions between phagocytes, NK cells, and the complement proteins are examples of the many ways in which innate system players work together. **Only by cooperating with each other can the players on the innate system team respond quickly and strongly to an invasion.**

A PROPORTIONAL RESPONSE

In reacting to an attack, our military tries to mount a response which is proportional to the threat. Such a response insures that, on the one hand, resources will not be wasted by overreacting, and on the other, that the reaction will be strong enough to get the job done. The immune system is also set up to provide a proportional response to microbial invasions. For example, the number of macrophages engaged in battle depends on the size of the attack – and the amount of chemicals given off by macrophages to summon neutrophils or activate NK cells depends on how many macrophages are fighting. Consequently, the more serious the invasion, the more macrophages will be involved, and the more neutrophils and NK cells will be mobilized. Likewise, the larger a bacterial invasion is, the more "danger molecules" like LPS will be present at the battle scene. And the more LPS there is, the more NK cells will be activated to produce battle cytokines like IFN-γ – which help activate macrophages. Because the magnitude of the immune response is directly linked to the seriousness of the attack, "the punishment usually fits the crime."

HOW THE INNATE SYSTEM DEALS WITH VIRUSES

When viruses enter (infect) human cells, they take over the cells' machinery and use it to produce many more copies of the virus. Eventually, these newly made viruses burst out of the infected cells, and go on to infect other cells in the neighborhood. We have already discussed some of the weapons the innate system can use to defend against viruses when they are outside of cells. For example, proteins of the complement system can opsonize viruses for phagocytosis by macrophages and neutrophils. In addition, complement proteins can poke holes in enveloped viruses (e.g., HIV-1) by constructing membrane attack complexes on the virus's surface.

Although the innate system is quite effective against viruses when they are <u>outside</u> of cells, once viruses enter cells, the weapons the innate immune system can bring to bear are rather limited. NK cells and activated macrophages secrete cytokines like IFN-γ and TNF that in some cases can reduce the amount of virus that infected cells produce. Secreted TNF also can kill some virus-infected cells, and cells infected by certain viruses can be killed directly by NK cells or by activated macrophages. However, each virus-infected cell can produce thousands of new viruses, and many viruses mutate rapidly, enabling them to evolve defenses that can protect them from the weapons of the innate immune system. Consequently, **although complement proteins, professional phagocytes, and NK cells can help contain a viral infection, especially in the early stages, more potent weapons frequently are required to deal with virus-infected cells. This is probably the reason Mother Nature invented the** adaptive immune system – the subject of our next few lectures.

SUMMARY FIGURE

In this figure, I have summarized some of the concepts we discussed in this lecture. For clarity, I have chosen a macrophage as a representative of the professional phagocytes, a bacterium as an example of an invader that exists outside human cells, and a virus as an example of an invader which must enter a human cell to complete its life cycle. At the end of Lectures 3, 4, and 6, I will expand this figure to include the players from the adaptive immune system as they take the field.

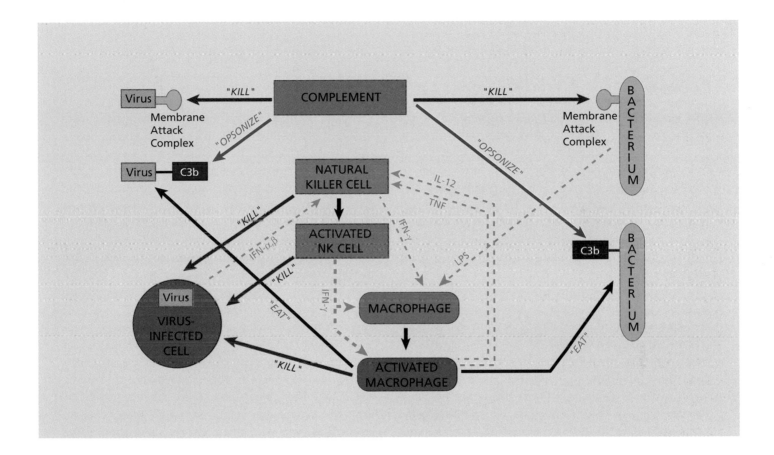

THOUGHT QUESTIONS

1. What is the fundamental difference in the way the complement system is activated by the alternative pathway and by the lectin activation pathway?

2. Why did Mother Nature make macrophages long-lived and neutrophils short-lived?

3. Give examples of the cooperation between players on the innate system team, and tell why this cooperation is important.

4. How do macrophages and natural killer cells tell friend from foe (i.e., how do they select their targets)?

5. Imagine a splinter has punctured your big toe, and that Gram-negative bacteria have invaded the tissues surrounding the splinter. Sketch the likely sequence of events in which the various players of the innate system team deal with this invasion.

6. Discuss how the innate system deals with a virus attack.

LECTURE 3

B Cells and Antibodies

REVIEW

Let's quickly review the material we covered in the last lecture. We talked about the complement system of proteins, and how complement fragments can function as "poor man's antibodies" to tag invaders for ingestion by professional phagocytes. In addition, complement fragments can act as chemoattractants to help recruit phagocytic cells to the battle site. Finally, the complement proteins can participate in the construction of membrane attack complexes that can puncture and destroy invading pathogens.

Complement proteins are present in high concentrations in the blood and in the tissues, so they are always ready to go. Activation by the "alternative" (spontaneous) pathway simply requires that a complement protein fragment, C3b, bind to an amino or hydroxyl group on an invader. Because these chemical groups are ubiquitous, the default option in this system is death: any surface that is not protected against binding by complement fragments will be targeted for destruction. Fortunately, there are multiple mechanisms which protect human cells from complement attack.

In addition to the alternative activation pathway, which can be visualized as "grenades" going off randomly here and there, we discussed a second pathway for activating the complement system that is more directed: the lectin activation pathway. In this system, a protein called mannose-binding lectin attaches to carbohydrate molecules that make up the cell walls of common pathogens. Then, a protein that is bound to the mannose-binding lectin sets off the complement chain reaction on the surface of the invader. So the mannose-binding lectin acts as a "guidance system" which targets the complement "bombs" to invaders that have distinctive carbohydrate molecules on their surfaces.

We also talked about two professional phagocytes: macrophages and neutrophils. In tissues, macrophages have a relatively long lifetime. This makes sense because macrophages act as sentinels that patrol the periphery. If they find an invader, they become "activated." In this activated state, they can present antigens to T cells, they send signals that recruit other immune system cells to help in the struggle – and they become vicious killers.

In contrast to sentinel macrophages, which reside beneath the surface of all the parts of our body that are exposed to the outside world, most neutrophils can be found in the blood – where they are "on call" in case of attack. Whereas macrophages are quite versatile, neutrophils mainly do one thing – kill. Neutrophils use cellular adhesion molecules to exit blood vessels at sites of inflammation, and as they exit, they are activated to become killers. Fortunately, these cells only live about five days. This limits the damage they can do to healthy tissues once an invader has been vanquished. On the other hand, if the attack is prolonged, there are plenty more neutrophils that can exit the blood and help out. Indeed, neutrophils represent about 70% of the circulating white blood cells.

The natural killer cell is another player on the innate team which is on call from the blood. These cells are a cross between a killer T cell and a helper T cell. NK cells resemble helper T cells in that they can secrete cytokines which affect the function of both the innate and the adaptive immune systems. And like CTLs, natural killer cells can destroy infected cells. However, in contrast to CTLs, which select their targets by surveying peptides displayed by class I MHC molecules, NK cells specialize in killing cells that don't express class I MHC molecules – especially "stressed" cells that have lost class I MHC expression.

How the Immune System Works, Fourth Edition. Lauren Sompayrac. © 2012 John Wiley & Sons, Ltd. Published 2012 by John Wiley & Sons, Ltd.

REVIEW (continued)

The innate system is programmed to react to "danger signals" that are characteristic of commonly encountered pathogens or pathogen-infected cells. Phagocytes, natural killer cells, and the complement proteins can attack immediately, because these weapons are already in place. As the battle continues, cooperation between these players increases to strengthen the defense, and signals given off by the innate system recruit even more defenders from the blood stream. By working together, members of the innate system team provide a fast and effective response to common invaders.

The innate system also plays a crucial role in alerting the adaptive immune system to danger. In fact, as we discuss the adaptive immune system, you will want to be on the lookout for interactions between the innate and adaptive systems. I think you'll soon appreciate that, although its rapid response is crucial for our survival, the innate system does much more than just react quickly.

Microbes such as bacteria and viruses are always mutating. Just as mutations in bacteria can render them resistant to certain antibiotics, mutations also can change microbes in ways that make them better able to resist immune defenses. When this happens, the immune system must "adapt" by producing new counter-weapons. Otherwise, the mutated microbe may take over. Indeed, a chess match has been going on for millions of years in which the immune systems of animals constantly have been "upgraded" in response to novel weapons fielded by microbial attackers. The most striking upgrade of the immune system began about 200 million years ago, when, in fish, evolution led to the precursor of what might be called the "ultimate defense" – a system so adaptable that, in principle, it can protect against any possible invader. This defense, the adaptive immune system, has reached its most sophisticated form in humans. Indeed, without an immune system which can recognize and adapt to deal with unusual invaders, human life would not be possible.

In this lecture, we will focus on one of the most important components of the adaptive immune system: the B cell. Like all the other blood cells, B cells are born in the bone marrow, where they are descended from stem cells. About one billion B cells are produced each day during the entire life of a human, so even old guys like me have lots of freshly made B cells. During their early days in the marrow, B cells select gene segments coding for the two proteins that make up their B cell receptors (BCRs), and these receptors then take up their positions on the surface of the B cell. The antibody molecule is almost identical to the B cell receptor, except that it lacks the protein sequences at the tip of the heavy chain which anchor the BCR to the outside of the cell. Lacking this anchor, the antibody molecule is exported out of the B cell (is secreted), and is free to travel around the body to do its thing.

THE B CELL RECEPTOR

I want to tell you a little about the process of selecting gene segments to make a B cell receptor. I think you'll find it interesting – especially if you like to gamble. **The BCR is made up of two kinds of proteins, the heavy chain (Hc) and the light chain (Lc), and each of these proteins is encoded by genes that are assembled from gene segments.** The gene segments that will be chosen to make up the final Hc gene are located on chromosome 14, and each B cell has two chromosome 14s (one from Mom and one from Dad). This raises a bit of a problem, because, as we discussed earlier, each B cell makes only one kind of antibody. Therefore, because there are two sets of Hc segments, it is necessary to "silence" the segments on one chromosome 14 to keep a B cell from making two different Hc proteins. Of course, Mother Nature could have chosen to make one chromosome a "dummy," so that the other would always be the one that was used – but she didn't. That would have been too boring. Instead, she came up with a much sweeter scheme, which I picture as a game of cards with the two chromosomes as players. It's a game of "winner takes all," in which each player tries to rearrange its cards (gene segments) until it finds an arrangement that works. The first player to do this wins.

You remember from the first lecture that the finished heavy chain protein is assembled by pasting together four separate gene segments (V, D, J, and C), and that lined up along chromosome 14 are multiple, slightly different copies of each kind of segment.

The players in this card game first choose one each of the possible D and J segments, and these are joined together by deleting the DNA sequences in between them. Then one of the many V segments is chosen, and this "card" is joined to the DJ segment, again by deleting the DNA in between. Right next to the rearranged J segment is a string of gene segments (C_M, C_D, etc.) that code for various constant regions. By default, the constant regions for IgM and IgD are used to make the BCR, just because they are first in line. Immunologists call these joined-together gene segments a "gene rearrangement," but it is really more about cutting and pasting than rearranging. Anyway, the result is that the chosen V, D, and J segments and the constant region segments all end up adjacent to each other on the chromosome.

Next, the rearranged gene segments are tested. What's the test? As you know, protein translation stops when the ribosome encounters one of the three stop codons, so if the gene segments are not joined up just right (in frame), the protein translation machinery will encounter a stop codon and terminate protein assembly somewhere in the middle of the Hc. If this happens, the result is a useless little piece of protein. In fact, you can calculate that each player only has about one chance in nine of assembling a winning combination of gene segments that will produce a full-length Hc protein. Immunologists call such a combination of gene segments a "productive rearrangement." If one of the chromosomes that is playing this game ends up with a productive rearrangement, that chromosome is used to construct the winning Hc protein. This heavy chain protein is then transported to the cell surface, where it signals to the losing chromosome that the game is over. Exactly how the signal is sent and how it stops the rearrangement of gene segments on the other chromosome remain to be discovered, although it is thought to have something to do with changing the conformation of the cell's DNA so that it no longer is accessible to the cut-and-paste machinery.

Since each player only has about a one in nine chance of success, you may be wondering what happens if both chromosomes fail to assemble gene segments that result in a productive rearrangement. Well, the B cell dies. That's right, it commits suicide! It's a high-stakes game, because a B cell that cannot express a receptor is totally useless.

If the heavy chain rearrangement is productive, the baby B cell proliferates for a bit, and then the light chain players step up to the table. The rules of their game are similar to those of the heavy chain game, but there is a second test which must be passed to win: the completed heavy and light chain proteins must fit together properly to make a complete antibody. If the B cell fails to productively rearrange heavy and light chains, or if the Hcs and Lcs don't match up correctly, the B cell commits suicide. So the result of this contest is that **every mature B cell produces one and only one kind of BCR or antibody, made up of one and only one kind of Hc and Lc. However, because a mix and match strategy is used to make the final Hc and Lc genes of each B cell, the receptors on different B cells are so diverse that collectively, our B cells can probably recognize any organic molecule that could exist.** When you consider how many molecules that might be, the fact that a simple scheme like this can create such diversity is truly breathtaking.

HOW THE BCR SIGNALS

Immunologists call the antigen that a given B cell's receptors recognize its "cognate" antigen, and the tiny region of the cognate antigen that a BCR actually binds to is called its "epitope." For example, if a B cell's cognate antigen happens to be a protein on the surface of the flu virus, the epitope will be the part of that protein (usually six to twelve amino acids) to which the BCR binds. When the BCR recognizes the epitope for which it is matched, it must signal this recognition to the nucleus of the B cell, where genes involved in activating the B cell can be turned on or off. But how does this BCR "antenna" send a signal to the nucleus that it has found its epitope? At first sight it would appear that this could be a bit of a problem, because, as you can see from this figure, the part of the heavy chain that extends through the cell membrane into the interior of the cell is only a few amino acids in length – way too short to do any serious signaling.

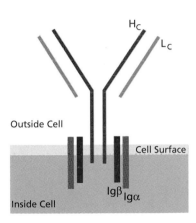

To make it possible for the external part of the BCR to signal what it has seen, B cells are equipped with two accessory proteins, Igα and Igβ, which associate with the heavy chain protein and protrude into the inside of the cell. Thus, **the complete B cell receptor really has two parts: the Hc/Lc part outside the cell that recognizes the antigen but can't signal, and the Igα and Igβ proteins that can signal, but which are totally blind to what's going on outside the cell.**

To generate an activation signal, many BCRs must be brought close together on the surface of the B cell. When BCRs are clustered like this, immunologists say they are "crosslinked" – although the receptors really are not linked together. B cell receptors can be clustered when they bind to an epitope that is repeated many times on a single antigen (e.g., a protein in which a sequence of amino acids is repeated many times).

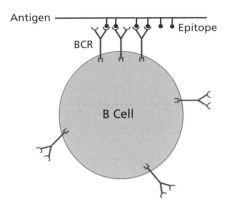

Crosslinking of BCRs also can result when BCRs bind to epitopes on individual antigens that are close together on the surface of an invader. Indeed, the surfaces of most bacteria, viruses, and parasites are composed of many copies of a few different proteins. So if a B cell's receptors recognize an epitope on one of these proteins, lots of BCRs can be clustered. In fact, the requirement for crosslinking is one way B cells focus on common enemies. Finally, B cell receptors can also be brought together by binding to epitopes on antigens that are clumped together (e.g., a clump of proteins). Regardless of how it is accomplished, crosslinking of B cell receptors is essential for B cell activation. Here's why.

The tails of the Igα and Igβ signaling molecules interact with enzymes inside the cell. When enough of these interactions are concentrated in one region, an enzymatic chain reaction is initiated which sends a message to the nucleus of the cell saying, "BCR engaged." So the trick to sending this message is to get lots of Igα and Igβ molecules together – and that's exactly what crosslinking of B cell receptors does. **The clustering of BCRs brings enough Igα and Igβ molecules together to set off the chain reaction that sends the "BCR engaged" signal. So BCR crosslinking is key.** Each B cell has about 100 000 BCRs on its surface, so there are plenty of B cell receptors to be clustered.

You remember from the last lecture that fragments of complement proteins (e.g., C3b) can bind to (opsonize) invaders. This tag indicates that the invader has been recognized as dangerous by the innate immune system, and invites innate system players such as macrophages to destroy the opsonized invader. It turns out that antigens opsonized by complement fragments also can alert the adaptive immune system. Here's how.

In addition to the B cell receptor and its associated signaling molecules, there is another protein on the surface of a B cell that can play an important role in signaling. This protein is a receptor that can bind to complement fragments which are decorating an invader. Consequently, for an opsonized antigen, there are two receptors on a B cell that can bind to the antigen: the BCR which recognizes a specific epitope on the antigen, and the complement receptor that recognizes the "decorations." When this happens, the opsonized antigen acts as a "clamp" that brings the BCR and the complement receptor together on the surface of the B cell.

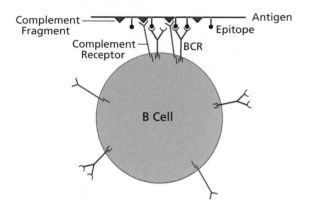

When the BCR and the complement receptor are brought together in this way by opsonized antigen, the signal that the BCR sends is amplified greatly. What this means in practice is that the number of BCRs that must be clustered to send the "receptor engaged" signal to the nucleus is decreased at least 100-fold. **Because the complement receptor can have such a dramatic effect on signaling, it is called a "co-receptor."** The function of this co-receptor is especially important during the initial stages of an attack, when the amount of antigen available to crosslink B cell receptors is limited. **Recognition of opsonized invaders by the B cell co-receptor also serves to make B cells exquisitely sensitive to antigens that the innate system has identified as being dangerous. This is an excellent example of the "instructive" function of the innate system. Indeed, the decision on whether an invader is dangerous or not is usually made by the innate, not the adaptive system.**

HOW B CELLS ARE ACTIVATED

To produce antibodies, B cells must first be activated. Most B cells have never encountered their cognate antigen, and these cells are called "naive" or "virgin" B cells. An example would be a B cell that can recognize the smallpox virus, but which happens to reside in a human who has never been exposed to smallpox. In contrast, B cells that have encountered their cognate antigen and have been activated are called "experienced." There are two ways that naive B cells can be activated to defend us against invaders. One is completely dependent on the assistance of helper T cells (T cell-dependent activation), and the second is more or less independent of T cell help (T cell-independent activation).

Activation of a naive B cell requires two signals. The first is the clustering of the B cell's receptors and their associated signaling molecules. However, just having its receptors crosslinked is not enough to fully activate a B cell – a second signal is required. Immunologists call this the "co-stimulatory" signal. In T cell-dependent activation, this second signal is supplied by a helper T cell. The best studied co-stimulatory signal involves direct contact between a B cell and a helper T (Th) cell. On the surface of activated Th cells are proteins called CD40L. When CD40L plugs into (ligates) a protein called CD40 on the surface of a B cell, the co-stimulatory signal is sent, and if the B cell's receptors have been crosslinked, the B cell is activated.

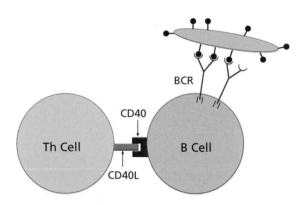

The interaction between these two proteins, CD40 and CD40L, is clearly very important for B cell activation. Humans who have a genetic defect in either of these proteins are unable to mount a T cell-dependent antibody defense.

In response to certain antigens, virgin B cells can also be activated with little or no T cell help, and this mode of activation is termed T cell-independent. What these antigens have in common is that they have repeated epitopes which can crosslink a ton of B cell receptors. A good example of such an antigen is a carbohydrate of the type found on the surface of many bacterial cells. A carbohydrate molecule is made up of many repeating units, much like beads on a string. If each "bead" is recognized by the BCR as its epitope, the string of beads can bring together many, many BCRs.

The crosslinking of such a large number of BCRs can partially substitute for co-stimulation by CD40L, and can cause a B cell to proliferate. But to be fully activated and produce antibodies, a naive B cell must receive a second signal. For T cell-independent activation, this second key is an unambiguous "danger signal" – a clear indication that an attack is on. One such signal is the recognition by the B cell of molecular patterns which are characteristic of certain bacteria and parasites. We will talk more about "pattern recognition receptors" in the next lecture. What is important for this discussion is that if a B cell has BCRs that can recognize a molecule with repeated epitopes like, for example, your own DNA, it may proliferate, but fortunately, no anti-DNA antibodies will be produced. The reason is that your immune system is not engaged in a battle with your own DNA, so there will be no danger signals to provide the necessary co-stimulation. On the other hand, if the innate immune system is battling a bacterial infection, and a B cell's receptors recognize a carbohydrate antigen with repeated epitopes on the surface of the bacterial invader, that B cell <u>will</u> produce antibodies – because danger signals from the battle field can supply the second key needed for complete B cell activation. Of course, as is true of T cell-dependent activation, **T-cell independent activation is antigen specific: only those B cells whose receptors recognize the repeated epitope will be activated.**

One advantage of T cell-independent activation is that B cells can jump right into the fray without having to wait for helper T cells to be activated. The result is a speedy antibody response to those invaders that can activate B cells independent of T cell help. But there is something else important going on here. Helper T cells only recognize protein antigens – the peptides presented by class II MHC molecules – so if all B cell activation required T cell help, the entire adaptive immune system would be focused on proteins. This wouldn't be so great, because many of the most common invaders have carbohydrates or fats on their surface that are <u>not</u> found on the surface of human cells. Consequently, these carbohydrates and fats make excellent targets for recognition by the immune system. So **by allowing some antigens to activate B cells without T cell help, Mother Nature did a wonderful thing: she increased the universe of antigens that the adaptive immune system can react against to include not only proteins, but carbohydrates and fats as well.**

In addition to T cell-dependent and T cell-independent activation of B cells, there is another, "unnatural" way that B cells can be activated. In this case the antigen, usually called a mitogen, binds to molecules on the B cell surface that are <u>not</u> B cell receptors, clustering these molecules. When this happens, BCRs that are associated with these molecules also can be clustered. In contrast to T cell-dependent and T cell-independent activation, this "polyclonal" activation does not depend on the cognate antigen that is recognized by the BCR – the BCR just comes along for the ride. In this way, many different B cells with many different specificities can be activated by a single mitogen. Indeed, mitogens are favorite tools of immunologists, because they can be used to activate a lot of B cells simultaneously, making it easier to study events that take place during activation.

One example of a mitogen is the highly repetitive structure that makes up the surface of certain parasites. During a parasitic infection, the molecules that make up these structures can bind to receptors (mitogen receptors) on the surface of B cells and cluster them – and when the mitogen receptors are brought together in this way, the cell's BCRs also are clustered. The result is polyclonal activation of B cells. But why would the immune system want to react to a parasitic attack by activating B cells whose BCRs do not even recognize the parasite? The answer is that this is <u>not</u> something the immune system was designed to do! By activating a bunch of B cells that will produce irrelevant antibodies, the parasite seeks to distract the immune system from focusing on the job at hand – destroying the parasitic invader. So **polyclonal activation of B cells by a mitogen actually is an example of the immune system gone wrong** – a subject we will discuss at length in another lecture.

Once B cells have been activated, and have proliferated to build up their numbers, they are ready for the next stage in their life: maturation. Maturation can be divided roughly into three steps: "class switching" in which a B cell can change the class of antibody it produces; "somatic hypermutation," in which the rearranged genes for the B cell receptor can undergo mutation and selection that can increase the affinity of the BCR for its cognate antigen; and the "career decision" during which the B cell decides whether to become an antibody factory (a plasma cell) or a memory B cell. The exact order of these maturation steps varies, and some B cells may skip one or more steps altogether.

CLASS SWITCHING

When a virgin B cell is first activated, it produces mainly IgM antibodies – the default antibody class. B cells also can produce IgD antibodies. However, IgD antibodies represent only a tiny fraction of the circulating antibodies in a human, and it is unclear whether they actually perform any significant function in the immune defense. You remember that an antibody's class is determined by the constant (Fc) region of its heavy chain – the "tail" of the antibody molecule, if you will. Interestingly, the same heavy chain messenger RNA (mRNA) is used to make both IgM and IgD, but the mRNA is spliced one way to yield an M-type constant region and another way to produce a D-type constant region.

As a B cell matures, it has the opportunity to change the class of antibody it makes to one of the other antibody classes: IgG, IgE, or IgA. Located just next to the gene segment on chromosome 14 that encodes the constant region for IgM are the constant region segments for IgG, IgE, and IgA. So all that a B cell has to do to switch its class is to cut off the IgM constant region DNA and paste on one of the other constant regions (deleting the DNA in between). Special switching signals that allow this cutting and pasting to take place are located between constant region segments on chromosome 14. For example, here's what happens when a B cell switches from an IgM constant region (C_M in this drawing) to an IgG constant region (C_G):

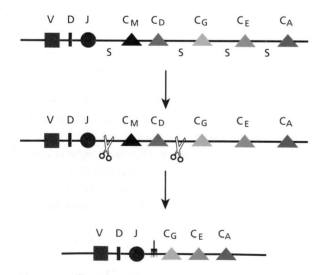

The net result of this switching is that although the part of the antibody that binds to the antigen (the Fab region) remains the same, the antibody gets a new Fc region. This

is an important change, because it is the constant region which determines how the antibody will function.

ANTIBODY CLASSES AND THEIR FUNCTIONS

Let's take a look at the four main classes of antibodies: IgM, IgA, IgG, and IgE. As you will see, because of the unique structure of its constant region, each antibody class is particularly well suited to perform certain duties.

IgM antibodies

IgM antibodies were the first class of antibodies to evolve, and even "lower" vertebrates (my apologies to the animal rights folks) have adaptive immune systems that produce IgM antibodies. So it makes sense that in humans, **when naive B cells are first activated, they mainly make IgM antibodies.** You may remember from the first lecture that an IgG antibody looks roughly like this:

Well, an IgM antibody is like five IgG antibody molecules all stuck together. It's really massive!

IgM Antibody

Producing IgM antibodies early during an infection actually is quite smart, because IgM antibodies are very good at activating the complement cascade (immunologists call this "fixing complement"). Here's how it works.

In the blood and tissues, some of the complement proteins (about 30 of them!) get together to form a big complex called C1. Despite its size, this complex of proteins cannot activate the complement cascade, because it's bound to an inhibitor molecule. However, if two or more C1 complexes are brought close together, their inhibitors fall off, and the C1 molecules can then initiate a cascade of chemical reactions that produces a C3 convertase. Once this happens, the complement system is in business, because, as you remember from the last lecture, a C3 convertase converts C3 to C3b, setting up an amplification loop that produces more and more C3b. So the trick to activating the complement system by this "classical" (antibody-dependent) pathway is to bring two or more of the C1 complexes together – and that's just what an IgM antibody can do.

When the antigen binding regions of an IgM antibody bind to an invader, C1 complexes can bind to the Fc regions of the antibody. Because each IgM antibody has five Fc regions close together (this is the important point), two C1 complexes can bind to the Fc regions of the same IgM antibody, bringing the complexes close enough together to set off the complement cascade. So the sequence of events is: the IgM antibody binds to the invader, several C1 molecules bind to the Fc region of the IgM antibody, and these C1 molecules trigger the complement chain reaction on the invader's surface.

The reason antibodies are so useful in this regard is that some clever bacteria have evolved coats which resist the attachment of complement proteins. However, B cells can produce antibodies which will bind to essentially any coat a bacterium might put on. Consequently, antibodies can extend the range of the complement system by helping attach complement proteins to the surface of wily bacteria. This is a nice example of the innate immune system (the complement proteins) cooperating with the adaptive immune system (IgM antibodies) to destroy an invader. In fact, the term "complement" was coined by immunologists when they first discovered that antibodies were much more effective in dealing with invaders if they were "complemented" by other proteins – the complement proteins.

The alternative (spontaneous) complement activation pathway that we talked about in the last lecture is totally non-specific: any unprotected surface is fair game. In contrast, the classical or antibody-dependent activation pathway is quite specific: only those antigens to which an antibody binds will be targeted for complement attack. In this system, the antibody identifies the invader, and the complement proteins do the dirty work.

Certain "subclasses" of IgG antibodies also can fix complement, because C1 can bind to the Fc region of these antibodies. However, IgG antibodies are real wimps, with only one Fc region per molecule. So bringing two C1 complexes close enough together to get things started requires that two molecules of IgG bind very close together on the surface of the invading pathogen – and this is likely to happen only when there is a lot of IgG around. So, early in an infection, when antibodies are just beginning to be made, IgM antibodies have a great advantage over IgG antibodies because they fix complement so efficiently. In addition, IgM antibodies are very good at "neutralizing" viruses by binding to them and preventing them from infecting cells. Because of these properties, IgM is the perfect "first antibody" to defend against viral or bacterial infections.

IgG antibodies

IgG antibodies come in a number of different subclasses that have slightly different Fc regions and therefore different functions. For example, one subclass of human IgG antibodies, IgG3, fixes complement better than any other IgG subclass. Likewise, the IgG1 subclass is very good at binding to invaders to opsonize them for ingestion by professional phagocytes. This is because macrophages and neutrophils have receptors on their surfaces that can bind to the Fc portion of IgG1 antibodies once those antibodies have bound to an invader.

Natural killer cells have receptors on their surface that can bind to the Fc region of IgG3 antibodies. As a result, IgG3 can form a bridge between an NK cell and its target by binding to the target cell (e.g., a virus-infected cell) with its Fab region, and to the NK cell with its Fc region. Not only does this bring the NK cell close to its target cell, but having its Fc receptors bound actually stimulates an NK cell to be a more effective killer. This process is called "antibody-dependent cellular cytotoxicity" (ADCC). In ADCC, the NK cell does the killing, but the antibody identifies the target.

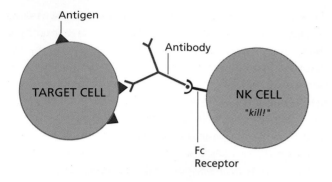

Like IgM antibodies, IgG antibodies also are very good at neutralizing viruses. However, IgG antibodies are unique in that they can pass from the mother's blood into the blood of the fetus by way of the placenta. This provides the fetus with a supply of IgG antibodies to tide it over until it begins to produce its own – several months after birth. This extended protection is possible because IgG antibodies are the longest-lived antibody class, with a half-life of about three weeks. IgM antibodies have a half-life of only about one day.

The "G" in IgG stands for "gamma," and IgG antibodies are sometimes called "gamma globulins." If there is a possibility that you have been exposed to an infectious agent, say hepatitis A virus, your doctor may recommend that you get a gamma globulin shot. These shots are prepared by pooling together antibodies from a large number of people, at least some of whom have been infected with hepatitis A virus, and are therefore making antibodies against the virus. The hope is that these "borrowed" antibodies will neutralize most of the virus to which you have been exposed, and that this treatment will help keep the viral infection under control until your own immune system can be activated.

IgA antibodies

Here's a question for you: what is the most abundant antibody class in the human body? No, it's not IgG. It's IgA. This is really a trick question, because I told you earlier that IgG was the most abundant antibody class in the blood – which is true. It turns out, however, that we humans synthesize more IgA antibodies than all the other antibody classes combined. Why so much IgA? Because IgA is the main antibody class that guards the mucosal surfaces of the body, and a human has about 400 square meters of mucosal surfaces to defend. These include the digestive, respiratory, and reproductive tracts. So although there aren't a lot of IgA antibodies circulating in the blood, there are tons of them protecting the mucosal surfaces. Indeed, about 80% of the B cells that are located beneath these surfaces produce IgA antibodies.

One reason IgA antibodies are so good at defending against invaders that would like to penetrate the mucosal barrier is that each IgA molecule is like two IgG molecules held together by a "clip."

IgA Antibody

The clipped-together tail structure of IgA antibodies is responsible for several important properties of this antibody class. This clip functions as a "passport" that facilitates the transport of IgA antibodies across the intestinal wall and out into the intestine. Moreover, this unique structure makes IgA antibodies resistant to acids and enzymes found in the digestive tract. Once inside the intestine, IgA antibodies can "coat" invading pathogens and keep them from attaching to the intestinal cells they would like to infect. In addition, whereas each IgG molecule has two antigen binding regions, the "dimeric" IgA molecule has four Fab regions to bind antigens. Consequently, dimeric IgA antibodies are very good at collecting pathogens together into clumps that are large enough to be swept out of the body with mucus or feces. In fact, rejected bacteria make up about 30% of normal fecal matter.

All together, these qualities make IgA antibodies perfect for guarding mucosal surfaces. Indeed, it is the IgA class of antibodies that is secreted into the milk of nursing mothers. These IgA antibodies coat the baby's intestinal mucosa and provide protection against pathogens that the baby ingests. This makes sense, because many of the microbes that babies encounter are taken in through their mouths – babies like to put their mouths on everything, you know.

Although IgA antibodies are very effective against mucosal invaders, they are totally useless at fixing complement, because C1 won't bind to an IgA antibody's Fc region. Again we see that the constant region of an antibody determines both its class and its function. This lack of complement-fixing activity is actually a good thing. If IgA antibodies could initiate the complement reaction, our mucosal surfaces would be in a constant state of inflammation in response to the pathogenic and non-pathogenic visitors that continuously assault our mucosal surfaces. And, of course, having chronically inflamed intestines would not be all that great. So IgA antibodies mainly function as "passive" antibodies that block the attachment of invaders to cells that line our mucosal surfaces, and usher these unwanted guests out of the body.

IgE antibodies

The IgE antibody class has an interesting history. In the early 1900s, a French physician named Charles Richet was sailing with Prince Albert of Monaco (Grace Kelly's father-in-law). The prince remarked to Richet that it was very strange how some people react violently to the toxin in the sting of the Portuguese man-of-war, and that this phenomenon might be worthy of study.

Richet took his advice, and when he returned to Paris, he decided, as a first experiment, to test how much toxin was required to kill a dog. Don't ask me why he decided to use dogs in his experiments. Maybe there were a lot of stray dogs around back then, or perhaps he just didn't like working with mice. Anyway, the experiment was a success and he was able to determine the amount of toxin that was lethal. However, many of the dogs he used in this first experiment survived, because they didn't receive the lethal dose. Not being one who would waste a good dog, Richet decided to inject these "leftovers" with the toxin again to see what would happen. His expectation was that these animals might have become immune to the effects of the toxin, and that the first injection would have provided protection (prophylaxis) against a second injection. You can imagine his surprise then, when all the dogs died – even the ones that received tiny amounts of toxin in the second injection. Since the first injection had the opposite effect of protection, Richet coined the word "anaphylaxis" to describe this phenomenon ("ana" is a prefix meaning "opposite"). Richet continued these studies on anaphylactic shock, and in 1913, he received the Nobel Prize for his work. I guess one lesson from this is that if a prince suggests you should study something, you might want to take his advice seriously!

Immunologists now know that **anaphylactic shock is caused by mast cells degranulating.** Like macrophages, mast cells are white blood cells that are stationed beneath all exposed surfaces (e.g., beneath the skin or the mucosal barrier). As blood cells go, mast cells are very long-lived.

They can survive for years in our tissues, lying in wait to protect against invaders. Recently, it has been learned that mast cells play a role in the innate defense against bacteria by phagocytosing opsonized bacteria, and by giving off cytokines that recruit neutrophils and other immune system cells to the site of a bacterial infection. However, the most important function of mast cells is to protect against infection by parasites that have penetrated the barrier defense. Stored safely inside mast cells are lots of granules that contain all kinds of pharmacologically active chemicals, the most famous of which is histamine. When a mast cell encounters a parasite, it dumps the contents of these granules (i.e., it "degranulates") onto the parasite to kill it. Unfortunately, in addition to killing parasites, mast cell degranulation also can cause an allergic reaction, and in extreme cases, anaphylactic shock. Here's how this works.

An antigen (e.g., the man-of-war toxin) that can cause an allergic reaction is called an allergen. On the first exposure to an allergen, some people, for reasons that are far from clear, make lots of IgE antibodies directed against the allergen. Mast cells have receptors on their surface that can bind to the Fc region of these IgE antibodies, and when this happens, the mast cells are like bombs waiting to explode.

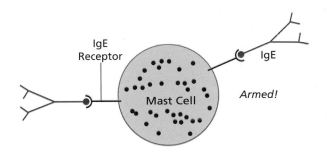

AFTER FIRST EXPOSURE

On a second exposure to the allergen, IgE antibodies that are already bound to the surfaces of mast cells can bind to the allergen. Because allergens usually are proteins with a repeating sequence, the allergen can crosslink many IgE molecules on the mast cell surface, dragging the Fc receptors together. This clustering of Fc receptors is similar to the crosslinking of B cell receptors in that bringing many of these receptors together results in a signal being sent. In this case, however, the signal says "degranulate," and the mast cell responds by dumping its granules into your tissues.

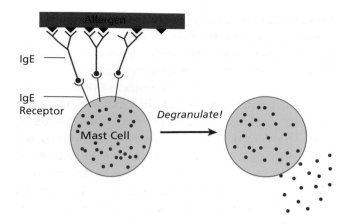

Histamines and other chemicals released from mast cell granules increase capillary permeability so that fluid escapes from the capillaries into the tissue – that's why you get a runny nose and watery eyes when you have an allergic reaction. This is usually a rather local effect, but if the toxin spreads throughout the body and triggers massive degranulation of mast cells, things can get very serious. In such a case, the release of fluid from the blood into the tissues can reduce the blood volume so much that the heart no longer can pump efficiently, resulting in a heart attack. In addition, histamine from the granules can cause smooth muscles around the windpipe to contract, making it difficult to breathe. In extreme cases, this contraction can be strong enough to cause suffocation. Most of us don't have to worry about being stung by a Portuguese man-of-war. However, some people make lots of IgE antibodies in response to bee toxin, and for those folks, a bee sting can cause fatal anaphylactic shock. Indeed, about 1,500 Americans die each year from anaphylactic shock.

This brings us to an interesting question: why are B cells allowed to switch the class of antibody they make anyway? Wouldn't it be safer just to stick with good old IgM antibodies? I don't think so. Let's suppose you have a viral infection of your respiratory tract, resulting in the common cold. Would you want to be stuck making only IgM antibodies? Certainly not. You'd want a lot of IgA antibodies to be secreted into the mucus that lines your respiratory tract to bind up that virus, and remove it from your body. On the other hand, if you have a parasitic infection (worms, for example), you'd want IgE antibodies to be produced, because IgE antibodies can cause cells like mast cells to degranulate, making life miserable for those worms. So **the beauty of this system is that the**

different classes of antibodies are uniquely suited to defend against different invaders.

ANTIBODY CLASS	ANTIBODY PROPERTIES
IgM	Great complement fixer Good opsonizer First antibody made
IgA	Resistant to stomach acid Protects mucosal surfaces Secreted in milk
IgG	OK complement fixer Good opsonizer Helps NK cell kill (ADCC) Can cross placenta
IgE	Defends against parasites Causes anaphylactic shock Causes allergies

Now suppose Mother Nature could arrange to have your immune system make IgG antibodies when your big toe is infected, IgA antibodies when you have a cold, or IgE antibodies when you have a parasitic infection? Wouldn't that be elegant? Well, it turns out that this is exactly what happens! Here's how it works.

Antibody class switching is controlled by the cytokines that B cells encounter when switching takes place: certain cytokines or combinations of cytokines influence B cells to switch to one class or another. For example, if B cells class switch in an environment that is rich in IL-4 and IL-5, they preferentially switch their class from IgM to IgE – just right for those worms. On the other hand, if there is a lot of IFN-γ around, B cells switch to produce IgG3 antibodies that are very effective against bacteria and viruses. Or, if a cytokine called TGFβ is present during the class switch, B cells preferentially change from IgM to IgA antibody production – perfect for the common cold. So **to insure that the antibody response will be appropriate for a given invader, all Mother Nature has to do is to arrange to have the right cytokines present when B cells switch classes.** But how could she accomplish this?

You remember that helper T cells are "quarterback" cells which direct the immune response. One way they do this is by producing cytokines which influence B cells to make the antibody class that is right to defend against a given invader. To learn how Th cells know which cytokines to make, you'll have to wait for the next three lectures when we discuss antigen presentation and T cell activation and function. But for now, I'll just give you the bottom line: **in response to cytokines made by Th cells, B cells can switch from making IgM antibodies to producing one of the other antibody classes. As a result, the adaptive immune system can respond with antibodies tailor-made for each kind of invader – be it a bacterium, a flu virus, or a worm.** What could be better than that?!

SOMATIC HYPERMUTATION

As if class switching weren't great enough, there is yet another amazing thing that can happen to B cells as they mature. Normally, the overall mutation rate of DNA in human cells is extremely low – only about one mutated base per 100 million bases per DNA replication cycle. It has to be this low or we'd all end up looking like Star Wars characters with three eyes and six ears. However, in very restricted regions of the chromosomes of B cells – those regions that contain the V, D, and J gene segments – an extremely high rate of mutation can take place. In fact, mutation rates as high as one mutated base per 1000 bases per generation have been measured. We're talking serious mutations here! This high rate of mutation is called "somatic hypermutation," and it occurs after the V, D, and J segments have been selected – and usually after class switching has taken place. So **somatic hypermutation is a relatively late event in the maturation of B cells. Indeed, B cells that still make IgM antibodies usually have not undergone somatic hypermutation.**

What somatic hypermutation does is to change (mutate) the part of the rearranged antibody gene that encodes the antigen binding region of the antibody. Depending on the mutation, there are three possible outcomes: the affinity of the antibody molecule for its cognate antigen may remain unchanged, it may be increased, or it may be decreased. Now comes the neat part. It turns out that for maturing B cells to continue to proliferate, they must be continually re-stimulated by binding to their cognate antigen. Therefore, because those B cells whose BCRs have mutated to higher affinity are stimulated more easily (because their BCRs bind better), they proliferate

more frequently than do B cells with lower-affinity receptors. And because B cells with high-affinity receptors proliferate more frequently, the result of somatic hypermutation is that you end up with many more B cells whose BCRs have high affinity for their cognate antigen.

By using somatic hypermutation to make changes in the antigen binding region of a BCR, and by using binding and proliferation to select those mutations that have increased the BCR's ability to bind to antigen, B cell receptors can be "fine-tuned." The result is a collection of B cells whose receptors have a higher average affinity for their cognate antigen. This whole process is called affinity maturation.

So B cells can change their constant (Fc) region by class switching, and their antigen binding (Fab) region by somatic hypermutation – and these two modifications produce B cells that are better adapted to deal with invaders. Both of these changes are controlled by cytokines that are provided mainly by helper T cells. As a result, B cells that are activated without T cell help (e.g., in response to carbohydrates on the surface of a bacterium) usually don't undergo either class switching or somatic hypermutation.

B CELLS MAKE A CAREER CHOICE

The final step in the maturation of a B cell is the choice of profession. This can't be too tough, because a B cell really only has two fates to choose between: to become a plasma cell or a memory cell. **Plasma cells are antibody factories.** If a B cell decides to become a plasma cell, it usually travels to the spleen or back to the bone marrow, and begins to produce the secreted form of the BCR – the antibody molecule. Some plasma B cells can mass produce 2000 of these antibodies each second. However, as a result of this heroic effort, these plasma B cells only live for a few days. The fact that one plasma B cell can make so many antibody molecules enables the immune system to keep up with invaders like bacteria and viruses which multiply very quickly.

Although the B cell's other possible career choice – to become a memory B cell – may not be quite so dramatic as the decision to become a plasma cell, it is extremely important. It is the memory B cell that remembers your first exposure to a pathogen, and helps defend you against subsequent exposures. Immunologists haven't figured out how a B cell "chooses" to become either a memory cell or a plasma cell. However, they do know that the interaction between the co-stimulatory molecule, CD40L, on the surface of a helper T cell and CD40 on the B cell surface is important in memory cell generation. Indeed, **memory B cells are not produced when B cells are activated without T cell help.**

SUMMARY FIGURE

Our summary figure now includes the innate immune system from the last lecture plus B cells and antibodies.

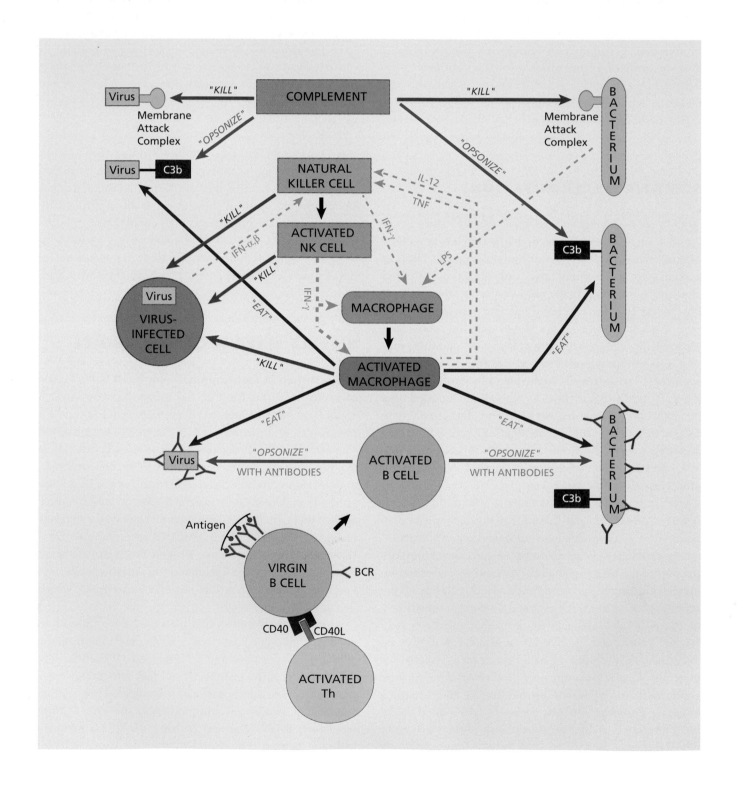

THOUGHT QUESTIONS

1. B cells are produced according to the principle of clonal selection. Exactly what does this mean?

2. Describe what happens during T cell-dependent activation of B cells.

3. Describe "fail-safe" systems that are involved in B cell activation.

4. How can B cells be activated without T cell help?

5. Why is T cell-independent activation of B cells important in defending us against certain pathogens?

6. Describe the main attributes of IgM, IgG, IgA, and IgE antibodies.

7. Why do class switching and somatic hypermutation produce B cells that are better able to defend against invaders?

8. Why do most mast cells wait until their second exposure to an allergen before they degranulate? Hint: Think about the timing.

LECTURE 4
The Magic of Antigen Presentation

REVIEW

In the last lecture, we discussed B cells and antibodies. Let's do a bit of review. A B cell's receptors function as the "eyes" of the cell, and actually have two parts: a recognition part (made up of the heavy and light chain proteins), and a signaling part (made up of two other proteins, $Ig\alpha$ and $Ig\beta$). The final genes that encode the recognition part are made by mixing and matching gene segments. The result is a collection of B cells with receptors so diverse that they probably can recognize any organic molecule in the universe. For these receptors to signal what they have seen requires that multiple BCRs be clustered (crosslinked). This crosslinking brings the $Ig\alpha$ and $Ig\beta$ signaling molecules that are associated with the heavy chains close together. And when enough $Ig\alpha$ and $Ig\beta$ molecules are clustered in this way, a threshold amount of enzymatic activity is reached, and the "receptor engaged" signal is sent to the nucleus of the B cell.

Activation of a virgin B cell requires two "keys." Crosslinking of the B cell's receptors is the first key. In addition, a second, "co-stimulatory" key also is required. This key usually is provided by a helper T cell, and involves cell–cell contact during which CD40L molecules on the surface of a helper T cell bind to CD40 proteins on the surface of a B cell. B cells can also be activated without T cell help. The first requirement for this T cell-independent activation is that a large number of the B cell's receptors must be crosslinked. This typically happens when the surface of an invader is made up of many copies of the antigen to which a B cell's receptors bind (its "cognate" antigen). Although the crosslinking of many B cell receptors is a requisite for T cell-independent activation of a naive B cell, it is not enough. A second, co-stimulatory signal also is needed. This co-stimulation is in the form of a "danger signal" which confirms that an authentic threat exists. By demanding that two keys must be supplied before a B cell can be activated, a fail-safe system is established that guards against inappropriate B cell activation.

IgM antibodies are the first antibodies produced by B cells in response to a pathogen that has not been encountered before. However, as a B cell matures, it can choose to produce a different class of antibody: either IgG, IgA, or IgE. This class switching does not change the antigen binding (Fab) region of the antibody. Consequently, the antibody recognizes the same antigen before and after its class has been switched. What does change during class switching is the Fc region of the heavy chain. This is the part of the molecule that determines how the antibody functions, with some functions being better suited to certain invaders than to others. Importantly, the choice of antibody class is determined by the cytokines present in the local environment of the B cell when switching takes place. So by arranging to have appropriate cytokines produced at the appropriate places, Mother Nature can insure that the right class of antibody is made to defend against a particular invader.

The other change that can take place as a B cell matures is somatic hypermutation. In contrast to class switching, in which the antibody gets a different Fc region, somatic hypermutation alters the antigen binding region of the antibody. Because the probability that a B cell will proliferate depends on the affinity of its BCR for antigen, the B cells which proliferate most will be those for which somatic hypermutation has increased the binding affinity of their BCRs. Consequently, somatic hypermutation and selection for proliferation result in a collection of B cells whose BCRs bind more tightly to the invader than did the original,

How the Immune System Works, Fourth Edition. Lauren Sompayrac. © 2012 John Wiley & Sons, Ltd. Published 2012 by John Wiley & Sons, Ltd.

Of all the concepts on which the immune system is based, perhaps the most elegant, and certainly the most unexpected, is antigen presentation: the concept of having one cell present protein fragments to another cell. As you will see, antigen presentation is central to the function of the adaptive immune system, with the cells that present antigen to T cells, the "antigen presenting" cells (APCs), playing a pivotal role. Let's begin by discussing the "billboards" on APCs that actually do the presenting: the class I and class II MHC molecules.

CLASS I MHC MOLECULES

The structures of both class I and class II MHC molecules have now been carefully analyzed, so we have a good idea of what both kinds of molecules look like. Class I molecules have a binding groove that is closed at both ends, so the small protein fragments (peptides) they present must fit within the confines of the groove (the "bun," if you will). Indeed, **when immunologists pried peptides from the grasp of class I molecules and sequenced them, they found that most of them are eight to eleven amino acids in length. These peptides are anchored at the ends, and the slight variation in length is accommodated by letting the peptide bulge out a bit in the center.**

Every human has three genes for class I MHC proteins (called HLA-A, HLA-B, and HLA-C), located on chromosome six. Because we have two chromosome sixes (one from Mom and one from Dad), we all have a total of six

class I MHC genes. Each class I HLA protein pairs with another protein called β2-microglobulin to make up the complete class I MHC molecule. In the human population, there are many, slightly different forms of the genes that encode the three class I HLA proteins. For example, there are at least 480 variants of the gene for the HLA-A protein, 800 different HLA-B genes, and 260 different HLA-C genes. The proteins encoded by these genes all have roughly the same shape, but they differ by one or a few amino acids. Immunologists call molecules that have many forms "polymorphic," and the class I HLA proteins certainly fit this description. In contrast, all of us have the same gene for the β2-microglobulin protein.

Because they are polymorphic, class I MHC molecules can have different binding motifs, and therefore can present peptides that have different kinds of amino acids at their ends. For example, some class I MHC molecules bind to peptides that have hydrophobic amino acids at one end, whereas other MHC molecules prefer basic amino acids at this anchor position. Since humans have the possibility of expressing up to six different class I molecules, collectively our class I molecules can present a wide variety of peptides. Moreover, although MHC I molecules are picky about binding to certain amino acids at the ends of the peptide, they are rather promiscuous in their selection of amino acids at the center of the protein fragment. As a result, **a given class I MHC molecule can bind to and present a large number of different peptides, each of which "fits" with the particular amino acids present at the ends of its binding groove.**

CLASS II MHC MOLECULES

Like class I molecules, class II MHC molecules (encoded by genes in the HLA-D region of chromosome six) are wildly polymorphic: within the human population many different versions of class II molecules exist. However, in contrast to class I MHC molecules, the binding groove of class II MHC molecules is open at both ends, so a peptide can hang out of the groove. As you might expect from this feature, peptides that bind to class II molecules are longer than those that occupy the closed groove of class I molecules – in the range of 13 to 25 amino acids. Further, for class II MHC molecules, the critical amino acids that anchor the peptides are spaced along the binding groove instead of being clustered at the ends.

ANTIGEN PRESENTATION BY CLASS I MHC MOLECULES

MHC I molecules are billboards that display on the surface of a cell, fragments of proteins manufactured by that cell. Immunologists call these "endogenous" proteins. These include ordinary cellular proteins like enzymes and structural proteins, as well as proteins encoded by viruses and other parasites that may have infected the cell. For example, when a virus enters a cell, it uses the cellular biosynthetic machinery to produce proteins encoded by viral genes. A sample of these viral proteins is then displayed by class I MHC molecules along with samples of all the normal cellular proteins. So in effect, the MHC I billboards advertise a "sampling" of all the proteins that are being made inside a cell. Almost every cell in the human body expresses class I molecules on its surface, although the number of molecules varies from cell to cell. Killer T cells (also called cytotoxic lymphocytes or CTLs) inspect the protein fragments displayed by class I MHC molecules. Consequently, almost every cell is an "open book" that can be checked by CTLs to determine whether it has been invaded by a virus or other parasite and should be destroyed. Importantly, after they have been on the surface for a short while, the MHC billboards are replaced by new ones – so the class I MHC display is kept current.

The way endogenous proteins are processed and loaded onto class I MHC molecules is very interesting.

When mRNA is translated into protein in the cytoplasm of a cell, mistakes are sometimes made. These mistakes can result in the production of useless proteins that don't fold up correctly. In addition, proteins suffer damage due to normal wear and tear. So to make sure our cells don't fill up with defective proteins, old or useless proteins are fed into protein-destroying "machines" in the cytoplasm that function rather like wood chippers. These protein chippers are called proteasomes, and they cut proteins up into small pieces (peptides). Most of these peptides are then broken down further into individual amino acids, which are reused to make new proteins. However, some of the peptides created by the proteasomes are carried by specific transporter proteins (TAP1 and TAP2) across the membrane of the endoplasmic reticulum (ER) – a large, sack-like structure inside the cell from which most proteins destined for transport to the cell surface begin their journey.

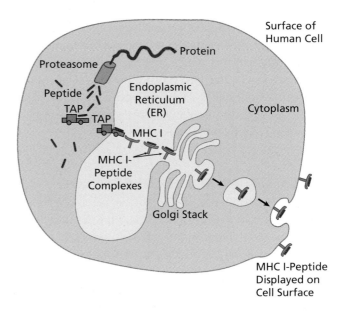

Once inside the ER, some of these peptides are chosen to be loaded into the grooves of class I MHC molecules. I say "chosen," because, as we discussed, not all peptides will fit. For starters, a peptide must be the right length – about nine amino acids. In addition, the amino acids at the ends of the peptide must be compatible with the anchor amino acids that line the ends of the groove of the MHC molecule. Obviously, not all of the "chips" prepared by the proteasome will have these characteristics, and those that don't are degraded or shipped back out of the ER into the cytoplasm. Once class I MHC molecules are loaded with peptides, they proceed to the surface of the cell for display. So **there are three main steps in preparing a class I display: generation of a peptide by the proteasome, transport of the peptide into the ER by the TAP transporter, and binding of the peptide to the groove of the MHC I molecule.**

In "ordinary" cells like liver cells and heart cells, the major function of proteasomes is to deal with defective proteins. So as you can imagine, the chippers in these cells are not too particular about how proteins are cut up – they just hack away. As a result, some of the peptides will be appropriate for MHC presentation, but most will not be. In contrast, in cells like macrophages that specialize in presenting antigen, this chipping is not so random. For example, binding of IFN-γ to receptors on the surface of a macrophage up-regulates expression of three proteins called LMP2, LMP7, and MECL1. These proteins replace three "stock" proteins which are part of the normal proteasome machinery. The result of this replacement is that the "customized" proteasomes now preferentially cut proteins after hydrophobic or basic amino acids. Why, you ask? Because the TAP transporter and MHC I molecules both favor peptides that have either hydrophobic or basic C-termini. **So in antigen presenting cells, standard proteasomes are modified so they will produce custom-made peptides, thereby increasing the efficiency of class I display.**

Proteasomes also are not too particular about the size of peptides they make, and since the magic number for class I presentation is about nine amino acids, you might imagine that the ER would be flooded with useless peptides that were either too long or too short. However, it turns out that the TAP transporter has the highest affinity for peptides that are eight to fifteen amino acids long. Consequently, the TAP transporter screens peptides produced by proteasomes, and preferentially transports those that have the right kinds of C-termini and which are approximately the correct length. Once candidate peptides have been transported into the ER, enzymes then trim off excess N-terminal amino acids to make the peptide the right size for binding to class I MHC molecules.

An important feature of this "chop it up and present it" system is that the majority of the proteins that are chopped up by proteasomes are newly synthesized proteins which are structurally defective. Consequently, most proteins are displayed on class I MHC molecules soon after they are produced. This means that you don't have to wait for proteins to wear out before they can be chopped up and presented – making it possible for the immune system to react quickly to an infection.

ANTIGEN PRESENTATION BY CLASS II MHC MOLECULES

Whereas class I MHC molecules are designed to present protein fragments to killer T cells, class II MHC molecules present peptides to helper T cells. And in contrast to class I MHC molecules, which are expressed on almost every kind of cell, class II molecules are expressed exclusively on cells of the immune system. This makes sense. Class I molecules specialize in displaying proteins that are manufactured <u>inside</u> the cell, so the ubiquity of class I molecules gives CTLs a chance to check most cells in the body for infection. On the other hand, class II MHC molecules function as billboards that advertise what is happening <u>outside</u> the cell to alert helper T cells to danger. Therefore, relatively few cells expressing class II are required for this task – just enough to sample the environment in various parts of the body.

The two proteins that make up the class II MHC molecules (called the α and β chains) are produced in the cytoplasm and are injected into the endoplasmic reticulum where they bind to a third protein called the invariant chain. **This invariant chain protein performs several functions. First, it sits in the groove of the MHC II molecule and keeps it from picking up other peptides in the ER.** This is important, because the ER is full of endogenous peptides that have been processed by proteasomes for loading onto class I MHC molecules. If these protein fragments were loaded onto class II molecules, then class I and class II MHC molecules would display the same kind of peptides: those made from proteins produced in the cell. Since the goal is to have class II MHC molecules present antigens that come from outside the cell, the invariant chain performs an important function by acting as a "chaperone" that makes sure "inappropriate suitors" (endogenous peptides) don't get picked up by MHC II molecules in the ER.

The invariant chain's second function is to guide class II MHC molecules out through the Golgi stack to special

vesicles in the cytoplasm called "endosomes." It is within endosomes that class II MHC molecules are loaded with peptides. I have to warn you, however, that when biologists don't understand something very well, they usually call it a "-some" – a suffix that means "body." And this is no exception, because it isn't clear yet exactly what goes on inside these endosomes.

The current thinking is that while class II MHC molecules are making their way from the ER to the endosome, proteins that are hanging around outside the cell are enclosed in a phagosome, and brought into the cell. This phagosome then merges with the endosome, and enzymes present in the endosome chop up the exogenous proteins from the phagosome into peptides. During this time, endosomal enzymes also destroy all of the invariant chain except the piece that is actually guarding the groove of the MHC molecule. Amazingly, although the exogenous proteins and the invariant chain are hacked to pieces by enzymes in the endosome, the class II MHC molecule itself remains unscathed. This is presumably because the MHC molecule is cleverly folded so that the enzymes cannot gain access to their favorite cleavage sites. Meanwhile, a cellular protein called HLA-DM, which also has traveled to the endosome, catalyzes the release of the remaining fragment of the invariant chain (called CLIP), allowing an exogenous peptide to be loaded into the now-empty groove of the class II MHC molecule. Finally, the complex of MHC plus peptide is transported to the cell surface for display.

This is probably more or less what happens, but the details are still fuzzy. The important point, however, is that **Mother Nature has arranged two separate loading sites and pathways for class I and class II MHC molecules. It is this separation of loading sites and pathways that allows the class I billboard to advertise what's going on inside the cell (for killer T cells), and the class II billboard to advertise what's happening outside (for helper T cells).**

Although the separation of class I and class II pathways is the "law," under certain experimental conditions, antigens taken up from outside a cell can be presented by class I MHC molecules. Such an unlawful use of the class I display has been termed "cross-presentation." To date, the rules governing cross-presentation have not been clearly defined, and it is not yet known whether, under normal circumstances, cross-presentation is an important feature of the human immune system.

ANTIGEN PRESENTING CELLS

Before a killer T cell can kill or a helper T cell can help, it must be activated. For this to happen, a T cell must recognize its cognate antigen presented by an MHC molecule on the surface of another cell. But this is not enough. It must also receive a second, co-stimulatory signal. Only certain cells are equipped to provide both class I and class II MHC display <u>and</u> co-stimulation. These are the professional antigen presenting cells (APCs).

Because the job of antigen presenting cells is to activate killer and helper T cells, these cells really should have been named "T cell-activating cells." This would have avoided confusion with the "ordinary" cells in the body, which cannot activate T cells, but which do use class I MHC molecules to present antigens made inside these cells to alert killer T cells. Does it seem to you that immunologists just like to make things confusing? I sometimes think so. Anyway, to keep this straight, just remember that **the term "antigen presenting cell" always refers to those special cells which can provide the high levels of MHC and co-stimulatory molecules required for T cell activation.**

Co-stimulation usually involves a protein called B7 on the surface of an antigen presenting cell that "plugs into" a protein called CD28 on the surface of a T cell.

Endoplasmic Reticulum (ER)

Cytoplasm

Surface of Human Cell

Invariant Chain-MHC II Complex

Invariant Chain

Golgi Stack

Clip

Endosome

Phagosome

Peptides

Protein

MHC II-Peptide Displayed on Cell Surface

Three types of antigen presenting cells have been identified: activated dendritic cells, activated macrophages, and activated B cells. It's interesting that all of these are white blood cells which start life in the bone marrow, migrate out to various sites in the body, and then must be activated before they can function as antigen presenting cells. New blood cells are made continuously, so APCs can be replenished as needed.

Activated dendritic cells

Dendritic cells have a characteristic, starfish-like shape, and they get their name from the word "dendrite," which is commonly used to describe the projections on nerve cells. The story about dendritic cells (DCs) is intriguing, because until not long ago, these cells were considered to be only a curiosity. However, it is now appreciated that these once obscure cells are the most important of all the antigen presenting cells – because dendritic cells can initiate the immune response by activating virgin T cells. Here's how this works.

The first DCs described were starfish-shaped, "Langerhans" cells that are found in the tissues just below the skin. However, dendritic cells have since been discovered all over the body. What is now clear is that dendritic cells are "sentinel" cells which take up positions beneath the barriers of epithelial cells that represent our first line of defense. In normal tissues (tissues that have not been infected), dendritic cells resemble wine tasters. Although they can take up about four times their volume of extracellular fluid per hour, they mostly just take it in and spit it back out. In this "resting" state, DCs express some B7 and relatively low levels of MHC molecules on their surface. As a result, resting dendritic cells are not very good at presenting antigen to T cells, especially to virgin T cells, which require extensive receptor crosslink-

ing by MHC-peptide complexes as well as powerful co-stimulation.

If there is a microbial invasion, and the tissues in which a dendritic cell resides become a battle site, the dendritic cell will become "activated." Immunologists have now identified two different kinds of signals which can activate dendritic cells. The first type of signal comes either from other immune system cells that are engaged in battle or from dying cells. For example, both neutrophils and macrophages give off tumor necrosis factor (TNF) when they are trying to destroy an attacker, and this battle cytokine can activate dendritic cells. In addition, cells that are being killed by invaders give off chemicals that can result in dendritic cell activation.

The second type of signal involved in the activation of antigen presenting cells comes from cellular receptors which recognize molecular "patterns" that are characteristic of broad classes of invaders. The "pattern recognition receptors" about which most is known are the Toll-like receptors (TLRs), and so far, eleven human TLRs have been discovered. Some are displayed on the surface of dendritic cells where they respond to invaders that are outside the cell. Other TLRs are found inside dendritic cells, and these receptors detect invaders which have already entered these cells.

Earlier, I mentioned one of the external receptors, TLR4, although I didn't call it by name. TLR4 is the receptor that dendritic cells and macrophages use to sense the presence of LPS – a component of the cell walls of many bacteria. TLR4 is anchored in the membrane that surrounds these antigen presenting cells, and it points outward to sense bacterial invaders in the external environment.

When invaders are phagocytosed, they end up in phago-lysosomes, where they eventually are destroyed. During this destruction, their "coats" are stripped off to reveal what is inside them. Some of the Toll-like receptors (e.g., TLR7 and TLR9) are located in the membranes that surround these phago-lysosomes, and these pattern-recognition receptors point inward into the phago-lysosome so that they can alert the cell to the presence of viruses or bacteria that have been phagocytosed. TLR7 detects the single-stranded RNA of viruses such as influenza and HIV-1, whereas TLR9 recognizes the double-stranded DNA of bacteria and herpes simplex virus.

There are two important features of the patterns recognized by Toll-like receptors. First, TLRs recognize general characteristics of classes of invaders – not just a single invader. For example, LPS is a component of the cell walls of many different bacteria, and single-stranded RNA is found in many viruses. Consequently, TLR4 can detect invasions by many different types of bacteria (those with LPS in their cell walls), and TLR7 alerts cells to attacks by many different viruses (those which carry their genetic information in the form of single-stranded RNA). So in contrast to BCRs and TCRs, which are specific for each invader, pattern-recognition receptors are "economical" in the sense that each one can identify many different pathogens.

The second important characteristic of the patterns which TLRs recognize is that they represent structural features which are so important to the pathogen that they cannot easily be altered by mutation to avoid detection. For example, TLR4 has evolved to recognize a region of the LPS molecule that is indispensable for constructing bacterial cell walls. Consequently, a bacterium would be in big trouble if that part of the LPS molecule were mutated to try to evade detection by TLR4.

Traveling dendritic cells

When a dendritic cell is activated by battle cytokines, chemicals given off by dying cells, ligation of its pattern-recognition receptors, or a combination of these signals, the lifestyle of this "wine taster" changes dramatically. No longer does the dendritic cell "sip and spit." Now it "swallows" what it has taken in. Typically, a dendritic cell remains in the tissues for about six hours after the attack begins, collecting battle antigens. At that point, phagocytosis ceases, and the activated dendritic cell leaves the tissues and travels through the lymphatic system to the nearest lymph node. It is its ability to "travel when activated" that makes the dendritic antigen presenting cell so special.

Inside a resting dendritic cell are large numbers of class II MHC molecules. When a resting DC is activated and starts to "mature" (as immunologists like to say), these "reserve" class II MHC molecules begin to be loaded with antigens from the battle scene. And by the time a DC reaches its destination – the trip usually takes about a day – these battle antigen-loaded class II MHC molecules will be prominently displayed on the surface of the cell. Also during its journey, the DC upregulates expression of its class I MHC molecules. Consequently, if the dendritic cell had been infected by a virus out at the battle scene, by the time it reaches a lymph node, fragments of viral proteins will be on display on the dendritic cell's class I MHC billboards. Finally, while traveling, the dendritic cell increases production of B7 co-stimulatory proteins. So by the time it reaches a lymph node, the mature dendritic cell has everything it needs to activate virgin T

cells: high levels of class I and class II MHC molecules loaded with the appropriate peptides, and plenty of B7 proteins.

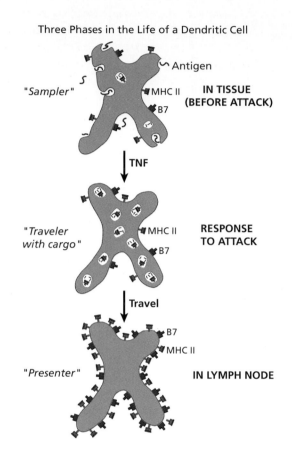

Three Phases in the Life of a Dendritic Cell

Now, why do you think it would be a good idea to have DCs, which wildly sample antigens out in the tissues, stop sampling when they begin their journey to a lymph node? Of course. Dendritic cells take a "snapshot" of what is happening on the "front lines," and carry this image to a lymph node – the place where virgin T cells congregate. There the traveling dendritic cells activate those virgin T cells whose T cell receptors recognize the invader that is "in the picture." The fact that battle cytokines such as TNF trigger the migration of DCs to a lymph node also makes perfect sense. After all, you want DCs to mature, travel to lymph nodes, and present antigen only if a battle is on.

Once a dendritic cell reaches a lymph node, it only lives for about a week. This short lifetime may seem strange at first. After all, this doesn't give a dendritic cell very long to meet up with the "right" virgin T cell that is circulating through the lymph nodes, looking for its cognate antigen. However, this short presentation life insures that dendritic cells carry snapshots of the battle which are up-to-date.

After a dendritic cell has been activated, but before it begins its travels, it produces special cytokines (chemokines) which encourage white blood cells called monocytes to leave the blood, enter the tissues, and become dendritic cells. Consequently, **activated dendritic cells recruit their own replacements**, and these newly recruited DCs carry fresh images of the battle to lymph nodes as the battle continues.

There is another reason for the short lifetime of dendritic cells. When a teacher disciplines a student, she follows the principle of "proportional response." For instance, if a student has left his homework at home, the teacher would not expel him for a month. No, she would respond in a way which is more appropriate to such a small offense. Likewise, it is important that the magnitude of an immune response be in proportion to the seriousness of the attack. Fortunately, the system was designed with this in mind, and the short lifetime of dendritic cells helps make this happen. Here's how.

During a microbial attack, the number of T cells which are activated will depend on the number of mature dendritic cells that bring news of the battle to nearby lymph nodes. For example, if the attack is weak, relatively few battle cytokines will be produced by warring macrophages, and only a small number of dendritic cells will be dispatched with their cargo. And because these DCs only live a short time once they reach the lymph node, only a limited number of T cells will be activated – just enough to deal with the small number of microbial invaders. On the other hand, if the infection is serious, many battle cytokines will be produced, many dendritic cells will be activated and travel to nearby lymph nodes, many more dendritic cells will be recruited from the blood, and many T cells will be activated. As a result of the dendritic cell's short lifetime, the number of dendritic cells in the lymph nodes at a given moment will reflect the current situation at the battle site, and the magnitude of the immune response will be proportional to the severity of the infection.

So **dendritic antigen presenting cells are sentinel cells that "sample" antigens out in the tissues. If there is an invasion, DCs become activated and travel to nearby lymph nodes. There they initiate the adaptive immune response by presenting antigen collected at the battle scene to virgin T cells. Activated DCs are short-lived, and the rapid turnover of these cells insures that the "pictures" they bring to a lymph node are continuously updated. Moreover, the number of dendritic cells dis-** patched from the tissues and the number of replacement dendritic cells recruited will depend on the severity of the attack. Consequently, the immune system is able to mount a response that is proportional to the danger posed by the invasion. Can you imagine a more ingenious system? I don't think so!

Dendritic cells are classified as members of the innate immune system because their receptors are "hard-wired," not adaptable like those of B and T cells. However, as I'm sure you now understand, dendritic cells actually function as a "bridge" between the innate and the adaptive systems.

Activated macrophages

Macrophages also are sentinel cells that stand guard over those areas of our body that are exposed to the outside world. They are very adaptable cells which can function as garbage collectors, antigen presenting cells, or ferocious killers, depending on the signals they receive from the microenvironment in which they reside. In a resting state, macrophages are good at tidying up, but they are not much good at antigen presentation. This is because macrophages only express enough MHC and co-stimulatory molecules to function as antigen presenting cells <u>after</u> they have been activated by battle cytokines such as IFN-γ, or by having their pattern-recognition receptors (e.g., their Toll-like receptors) ligated by invading pathogens.

So macrophages resemble dendritic cells in that they efficiently present antigen only when there is something dangerous to present. However, it is important to recognize that **dendritic antigen presenting cells don't kill, and macrophages don't travel.** Indeed, DCs can be pictured as "photojournalists" who don't carry weapons, and who take snapshots of the fighting, and who then leave the battlefield to file their stories. In contrast, macrophages are heavily armed soldiers who must stand and fight. After all, macrophages are one of our main weapons in the early defense against invaders. However, their lack of mobility raises an interesting question: What good is the activated macrophage's capacity to present antigen if it can't travel to lymph nodes where virgin T cells are located? Here's the answer.

Once they have been activated by dendritic cells, T cells exit the lymph nodes, circulate through the blood, and enter inflamed tissues to help with the battle. However, these "experienced" T cells must be continually restimulated. Otherwise, they think the battle has been won, and they go back to a resting state or die of neglect. That's where activated macrophages come in.

Macrophages act as "refueling stations" which keep experienced T cells "turned on" so they can continue to participate in the battle. So **mature dendritic cells activate virgin T cells, and activated macrophages mainly function to re-stimulate experienced T cells.**

Activated B cells

The third professional APC is the activated B cell. A virgin B cell is not much good at antigen presentation, because it expresses only low levels of class II MHC molecules and little or no B7. However, once a B cell has been activated, the levels of class II MHC molecules and B7 proteins on its surface increase dramatically. As a result, **an experienced B cell is able to act as an antigen presenting cell for Th cells.** B cells are not used as APCs during the initial stages of an infection, because at that time they are still naive – they haven't been activated. However, later in the course of the infection or during subsequent infections, presentation of antigen by experienced B cells plays an important role. Indeed, B cells have one great advantage over the other APCs: B cells can concentrate antigen for presentation. Here's how this works.

After a B cell's receptors have bound to their cognate antigen, the whole complex of BCR plus antigen is removed from the cell surface and dragged into the cell. There the antigen is processed, loaded onto class II MHC molecules, and transported back to the cell surface for presentation.

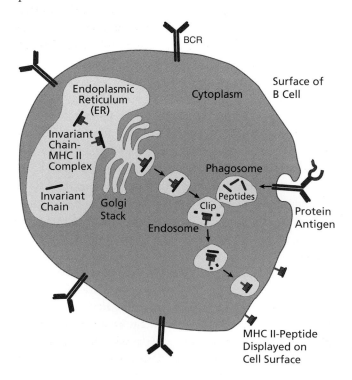

Because B cell receptors have such a high affinity for antigen, they act like "magnets," collecting antigen for presentation to Th cells. Since a threshold number of T cell receptors must be crosslinked by presented antigen before a Th cell can be activated, it is estimated that B cells have a 100- to 10 000-fold advantage over other APCs in activating helper T cells at times when there is relatively little antigen around. Presentation of antigen by B cells is also very fast. Less than half an hour elapses between the time antigen is captured by a B cell's receptors and the time it is displayed on the cell surface by class II MHC molecules.

In summary, **when an invader is first encountered, all the B cells which could recognize that particular invader are virgins, so the important APCs are activated dendritic cells. Then, while the battle is raging, activated macrophages on the front lines present antigen to warring T cells to keep them pumped up. Later, if this same invader is encountered again, experienced memory B cells left over from the first attack are the most important APCs – because they can get the adaptive immune response cranked up quickly by concentrating small amounts of antigen for presentation.**

NON-CLASSICAL MHC MOLECULES AND LIPID PRESENTATION

Class I and class II MHC molecules are called "classical" MHC molecules. So as you might expect, there also are "non-classical" MHC molecules. The best studied of these is the CD1 family of proteins. These non-classical MHC molecules resemble class I MHC molecules in that they consist of a long, heavy chain protein which is paired with the β2-microglobulin protein. However, in contrast to classical MHC molecules, which have grooves that are suitable to bind short peptides, the CD1, non-classical MHC molecules have evolved grooves which are designed to bind lipids. CD1 molecules can "sample" lipids from various compartments within a cell, and can present these molecules on the surface of antigen presenting cells, where they can activate T cells. Consequently, it has been postulated that these non-classical MHC molecules give T cells a way of surveying the lipid composition of cells, just as class I MHC molecules allow T cells to examine a cell's proteins.

For every rule in immunology there seems to be an exception, and the rule has been that T cells only recognize fragments of proteins presented by class I and class

II MHC molecules. Obviously, CD1 presentation of lipids to killer T cells is an exception to this rule. So far, however, it is not clear just how important CD1 presentation of lipids is for the immune defense. For example, killer T cells that recognize lipids produced by tuberculosis bacteria and presented by CD1 molecules have been isolated from patients with tuberculosis. However, it is not known how critical these killer T cells are in the defense against TB. Indeed, it is believed that the innate system is the primary defender against this pathogen. Because the importance of lipid recognition by T cells in defending us against invaders is not known at the present time, I will "stick to the rule" that T cells only recognize protein antigens. Be aware, however, that this may change as more research is done on CD1-presented lipids.

THE LOGIC OF CLASS I MHC PRESENTATION

To really appreciate why antigen presentation is one of Mother Nature's greatest inventions, we need to think a little about the logic behind this amazing activity. For starters, we need to ask the question: why bother with MHC presentation at all? Why not just let a T cell's receptors recognize unpresented antigen the way a B cell's receptors do? This is really a two-part question, since we are talking about two rather different displays: class I and class II. So let's discuss these one at a time.

Certainly **one reason for class I presentation is to focus the attention of killer T cells on infected cells, not on viruses and other pathogens that are outside our cells in blood and tissues.** So long as pathogens remain outside of our cells, antibodies can tag them for destruction by professional phagocytes, and can bind to them to prevent them from initiating an infection. Since each plasma B cell can pump out about 2000 antibody molecules per second, these antibodies are "cheap" weapons that deal quite effectively with extracellular invaders. However, once microbes enter a cell, antibodies can't get at them. When this happens, killer T cells – the high-tech, "expensive" weapons specifically designed to destroy infected cells – are needed. And the requirement that killer T cells recognize antigens presented by class I MHC molecules on infected cells insures that CTLs won't waste their time going after invaders which are outside of cells – where cheap antibodies usually can deal with them quite effectively.

In addition, **it would be extremely dangerous to have unpresented antigen signal T cell killing.** Imagine how terrible it would be if uninfected cells happened to have debris from dead viruses stuck to their surfaces, and killer T cells recognized this unpresented antigen and killed these "innocent bystander" cells. That certainly wouldn't do.

There's another reason why class I display is so important. **Most proteins made in a pathogen-infected cell remain inside the cell, and never make their way to the cell surface. So without class I display, many pathogen-infected cells would go undetected. In fact, part of the magic of the class I MHC display is that, in principle, every protein of an invading pathogen can be chopped up and displayed by class I MHC molecules for killer T cells to view.**

Finally, because their receptors recognize "native" antigens that have not been fragmented and presented, B cells actually are at a disadvantage. The reason is that most proteins must be folded in order to function properly. As a result of this folding, many targets (epitopes) that a B cell's receptors might recognize are unavailable for viewing – because they are on the inside of a folded protein molecule. In contrast, **when a protein is chopped up into short pieces and presented by class I MHC molecules, epitopes cannot be hidden from killer T cells.**

So the logic of class I MHC presentation is easy to understand, but why did Mother Nature make MHC molecules so polymorphic? After all, there are so many different forms in the human population that most of us inherit genes for six different class I molecules. Doesn't this seem a bit excessive? I mean, why not just let everybody express the same MHC I molecule?

Well, suppose we all did have just one gene for class I MHC proteins, and that it was the same for everyone. Now imagine what might happen if a virus were to mutate so that none of its peptides would bind to that single MHC I molecule. Such a virus could wipe out the entire human population, because no killer T cells could be activated to destroy virus-infected cells. So polymorphic MHC molecules give at least some people in the population a chance of surviving an attack by a clever pathogen.

On a more personal level, the fact that each of us has the possibility of "owning" up to six different class I MHC molecules increases the probability that we will have at least one class I MHC molecule into which a given pathogen's protein fragments will fit. Indeed, AIDS patients who have inherited the maximum number of different class I MHC molecules (six) live significantly longer than patients who have genes for only five or fewer different class I molecules. The thinking here is that as the AIDS virus mutates, having a larger number of different class I molecules increases the probability that mutated viral proteins can be presented.

THE LOGIC OF CLASS II MHC PRESENTATION

Okay, so class I MHC presentation makes a lot of sense. But what about class II presentation? At first glance, this "dual display" (class I and class II) by antigen presenting cells might seem overly complicated. What must be appreciated, however, is that many pathogens do not infect human cells; they are quite happy living and reproducing outside our cells in our tissues or in our blood. If antigen presenting cells could only display proteins made by pathogens that infect them, intelligence on many of the most damaging microbes would never reach the command centers in lymph nodes. By using class II MHC molecules to advertise a sampling of the total environment at the battle front, intelligence on all types of invaders can be made available to helper T cells.

But couldn't helper T cells just recognize unpresented antigen? After all, they aren't killers, so there isn't the problem of bystander killing. That's true, of course, but there is still a safety issue here. **Antigen presenting cells only present antigen efficiently when a battle is going on, and helper T cells are educated not to react to our own proteins. Consequently, both the helper T cell and the antigen presenting cell must "agree" that there has been an invasion before a helper T cell can be activated. By requiring that helper T cells only recognize presented antigen, Mother Nature guarantees that the decision to deploy the deadly adaptive immune system is not made by a single cell.**

Also, like class I molecules, class II molecules present small fragments of proteins. As a result, **the number of targets that a helper T cell can "see" during presentation far exceeds those available for viewing in a large, folded protein. The consequence of this expanded number of targets is a stronger and more diverse immune reaction in which many different helper T cells will be activated – helper T cells whose receptors recognize the many different epitopes that make up the antigens of an invader.**

MHC PROTEINS AND ORGAN TRANSPLANTS

In addition to their "natural" role in antigen presentation, MHC molecules also are important in the "unnatural" setting of organ and tissue transplantation. Transplantation studies actually began in the 1930s with experiments involving mouse tumors. In those days, tumors were usually induced by rubbing some horrible chemical on the skin of a mouse, and then waiting for a long time for a tumor to develop. Because it was so much trouble to make these tumors, biologists wanted to keep the tumor cells alive for study after the mouse had died. They did this by injecting some of the tumor cells into another, healthy mouse, where the cells would continue to grow. What they observed, however, was that the tumor cells only could be successfully transplanted when the two mice were from a strain of mice in which there had been a lot of inbreeding. And the more inbred the strain, the better the chance for survival of the transplant. This provided the impetus for the creation of a number of inbred mouse strains that immunologists depend on today. Just so you know, it takes over two years of constant breeding to produce a strain of mice that is truly inbred – a strain in which all the mice have essentially the same genetic makeup.

Once inbred mouse strains were available, immunologists began to study the transplantation of normal tissues from one mouse to another. Right away they noticed that if a small patch of skin from one mouse was grafted onto the skin of another mouse, this new skin retained its healthy pink color and continued to grow so long as the two mice were from the same inbred strain. In contrast, when this experiment was tried with mice that were not inbred, the transplanted skin turned white within hours (suggesting the blood supply had been cut off) and invariably died. Immunologists figured this immediate graft rejection must be due to some genetic incompatibility, because it did not occur with inbred mice that have the same genes. To identify the genes that are involved in "tissue compatibility" (histocompatibility), immunologists bred mice to create strains that differed by only a few genes, yet which were still incompatible for tissue transplants. Whenever they did these experiments, they kept identifying genes that were grouped in a complex on mouse chromosome seventeen – a complex they eventually called the "major histocompatibility complex" or MHC.

So the MHC molecules that we have been discussing in the context of antigen presentation are the very same molecules that are responsible for immediate rejection of transplanted organs. It turns out that killer T cells are particularly sensitive to MHC molecules that are "foreign," and when they see them, they attack and kill the cells that express them. Some of their favorite targets are the cells that make up the blood vessels contained within the donated organ. By destroying these vessels, CTLs cut off the blood supply to the transplanted organ, usually resulting in its death. It is for this reason that transplant surgeons try to match donors and recipients who have the same MHC molecules. However, finding such a match is difficult. Indeed, it is estimated that if you had access to organs contributed by 10 000 000 different individuals who were not related to you, the chance of your finding an organ in this collection that is an exact match to all your class I and class II MHC molecules would only be about 50%. So the diversity of MHC molecules, which is so important in protecting us from new invaders, creates a real problem for organ transplantation.

SUMMARY

Antigen presentation by MHC molecules is an elegant solution to a number of problems that face the immune system. Presentation by class I MHC molecules insures that killer T cells stay focused on infected cells, that innocent bystanders are not killed by mistake, and that a clever pathogen cannot hide in an infected cell by keeping all its proteins internal. MHC presentation of protein fragments greatly increases the universe of antigens that are available for killer T cells and helper T cells to recognize, because epitopes hidden in a folded protein are revealed. And because MHC molecules are so polymorphic, it is likely that at least some humans will have MHC molecules which can display protein fragments from any pathogen. Finally (and perhaps most importantly), helper T cells and killer T cells must recognize their cognate antigens presented by antigen presenting cells before they can be activated. This requirement for antigen presentation during activation sets up a fail-safe system in which the decision to activate the adaptive immune system always involves more than one cell.

Now that you understand how antigens are presented and why presentation by class I and class II MHC molecules is such a great idea, we need to turn our attention to the cells that are "looking at" these two kinds of display – the helper T cell and the CTL. How these cells react to presented antigen is the subject of our next lecture.

SUMMARY FIGURE

You will notice that our summary figure now includes antigen presenting cells with their MHC and B7 molecules.

THOUGHT QUESTIONS

1. Mother Nature uses "fail-safe technology" to prevent inappropriate activation of the immune system. Can you give several examples of this strategy?

2. Give several reasons why antigen presentation by class I MHC molecules is important for the function of the adaptive immune system.

3. Why does antigen presentation by class II MHC molecules make good sense?

4. Describe the different roles that activated dendritic cells, activated macrophages, and activated B cells play in the presentation of antigen during the course of an infection.

5. During their lifetimes, dendritic antigen presenting cells can be "samplers," "travelers," and "presenters." Describe what DCs are doing during each of these three stages.

6. Some peptides are presented more efficiently than others. What factors influence the efficiency of presentation by class I and class II MHC molecules?

LECTURE 5

T Cell Activation

REVIEW

In the last lecture we talked about MHC molecules and antigen presenting cells (APCs). Class I MHC molecules function as billboards that display what is going on inside a cell. For example, when a virus infects a cell, it uses that cell's biosynthetic machinery to produce viral proteins. Some of these proteins are cut up into small pieces (peptides) by the proteasome, and carried by the TAP transporters into the endoplasmic reticulum (ER). There the peptides are "interviewed" by class I molecules. Those that are about nine amino acids in length with appropriate amino acids at their ends are bound in the grooves of class I MHC molecules, and are transported to the surface of the cell. By scanning the MHC I–peptide complexes displayed there, killer T cells can "look into a cell" to determine whether it has been infected and should be destroyed.

Class II MHC molecules are also billboards, but they are designed to alert helper T cells that a battle is being waged. Class II molecules are assembled in the ER, just like class I molecules, but because invariant chain proteins occupy their binding grooves, class II molecules do not pick up peptides in the ER. Instead, the class II–invariant chain complex is transported out of the ER and into another cellular compartment called an endosome. There they meet up with proteins that have been taken into the cell by phagocytosis and cut up into peptides by enzymes. These peptides then replace the invariant chains that have been guarding the grooves of the class II molecules, and the MHC–peptide complexes are transported to the cell surface for display to Th cells. By this clever mechanism, class II molecules pick up peptides derived from proteins taken in from outside the cell, but avoid peptides derived from proteins made within the cell.

The display by MHC molecules of fragmented proteins has several advantages over a display of intact proteins. First, most viral proteins normally remain hidden inside an infected cell and are not found on the cell surface. So these proteins would never be seen by killer T cells unless they were advertised by class I MHC molecules. In addition, because protein folding can hide large portions of a protein from view, chopping a protein up into small peptides reveals many potential T cell targets that would be inaccessible in an intact protein. Consequently, MHC display greatly increases the probability that CTLs will recognize an infected cell and that helper T cells will be alerted to a microbial attack.

Before killer T cells or helper T cells can function, they must be activated, and it is the task of the antigen presenting cell to do the activating. The requirement for activation insures that T cells only spring into action when both the T cell and the antigen presenting cell agree that there has been an invasion. In addition to expressing class I and class II molecules, APCs also provide the co-stimulatory signals required for T cell activation. The most important antigen presenting cell during the initial stages of an attack is the dendritic cell, because this cell can activate virgin T cells. When a dendritic cell detects danger signals at the scene of the battle, it migrates with its cargo of "battle antigen" to a nearby lymph node. There, the dendritic cell uses class II MHC molecules to display fragments of proteins it has collected out in the tissues, and class I MHC molecules to display fragments of proteins made by viruses or bacteria that have infected the dendritic cell out at the battle site. In this way, the dendritic cell effectively takes a snapshot of what is going on at the front, carries it to the place

How the Immune System Works, Fourth Edition. Lauren Sompayrac. © 2012 John Wiley & Sons, Ltd. Published 2012 by John Wiley & Sons, Ltd.

where T cells are plentiful, and then does its "show and tell" thing to activate T cells.

Macrophages, activated by danger signals, also can function as antigen presenting cells. However, activated macrophages don't travel to lymph nodes to present antigen. They stay put in the tissues and battle invaders. Consequently, macrophages are most useful for presenting antigen after the adaptive immune system has been activated. At that time, activated macrophages out in the tissues can keep experienced T cells fired up, prolonging the time that they are effective in dealing with invaders.

Activated B cells are the third type of antigen presenting cell, but again, these cells aren't useful in initiating the adaptive response. The reason is that before B cells can function as antigen presenting cells, they must first be activated by helper T cells – and Th cells must wait to be activated by dendritic cells. So B cells don't get "certified" to be antigen presenting cells until after the adaptive immune response has already fired up. However, once activated, B cells have a great advantage over dendritic cells and macrophages: B cells can use their receptors as "antigen collectors" to concentrate small amounts of antigen for presentation to helper T cells. Consequently, relatively late in the initial infection or early in a subsequent infection by the same attacker, B cells play a major role as antigen presenting cells.

The innate immune system maintains large stockpiles of weapons. This makes sense because common invaders are attacking our bodies almost continuously, and the weapons of the innate immune system are useful against a wide variety of these "everyday" enemies. In contrast, only about one in a million B or T cells will have receptors that can recognize a given invader. So it would not be wise to stockpile B or T cells, because in our entire lifetime, we probably will never encounter an invader which a particular B or T cell could defend against. Indeed, **an important feature of the adaptive immune system is that its weapons are made on demand: only those B and T cells whose receptors can recognize the "invader *du jour*" are mobilized.** The first step in mobilizing these weapons is activation, and in this lecture, we're going to focus on how T cells are activated. What they do once they are activated will be the subject of the next lecture.

T CELL RECEPTORS

T cell receptors (TCRs) are molecules on the surface of a T cell that function as the cell's "eyes" on the world. Without these receptors, T cells would be flying blind with no way to sense what's going on outside. T cell receptors come in two flavors: $\alpha\beta$ and $\gamma\delta$. Each type of receptor is composed of two proteins, either α and β or γ and δ. Like the heavy and light chains of the B cell receptor, the genes for α, β, γ, and δ are assembled by mixing and matching gene segments. In fact, in B and T cells, the same proteins (RAG1 and RAG2) initiate the splicing of

gene segments by making double-stranded breaks in chromosomal DNA. As the gene segments are mixed and matched, a "competition" ensues from which each T cell emerges with either an $\alpha\beta$ or a $\gamma\delta$ receptor, but not both. Generally, all the TCRs on a mature T cell are identical – although there are exceptions to this rule.

TRADITIONAL T CELLS

Over 95% of the T cells in circulation have $\alpha\beta$ T cell receptors, and express either CD4 or CD8 "co-receptor" molecules (more about co-receptors in a bit). The $\alpha\beta$ receptors of these "traditional" T cells recognize a complex composed of a peptide and an MHC molecule on the surface of a cell, and a given T cell will have receptors that recognize peptides associated either with class I MHC molecules or with class II MHC molecules. Importantly, the **$\alpha\beta$ receptors of a traditional T cell recognize <u>both</u> the peptide and the MHC molecule.**

NON-TRADITIONAL T CELLS

In addition to traditional T cells, several kinds of "non-traditional" T cells have been discovered. T cells which have $\gamma\delta$ receptors can be considered to be non-traditional because, in contrast to traditional T cells, most $\gamma\delta$ T cells do not express either the CD4 or CD8 co-receptor molecules. T cells with $\gamma\delta$ receptors are most abundant in areas like the intestine, the uterus, and the tongue which are in contact with the outside world. Interestingly, mice have lots of γδ T cells in the epidermal layer of their skin, but humans do not. This serves to remind us that so far as the immune system is concerned, humans are not just big mice. After all, human and mouse lineages diverged roughly 65 million years ago, and humans are relatively large animals which can live a long time. In contrast, mice are small and short-lived. In fact, an "elderly" mouse is about two years old. Consequently, we would predict that, although similar, the immune systems which evolved to protect these two, very different animals, would be different. And they are.

Although αβ TCRs are thought to be about as diverse as BCRs, γδ receptors are much less diverse. Moreover, the receptors of γδ T cells in the tongue and uterus tend to favor certain gene segments during rearrangement, whereas γδ receptors in the intestine prefer other combinations of gene segments. The thinking here is that, **like players on the innate immune system team, γδ T cells stand watch on the "front lines," and have receptors which are "tuned" to recognize invaders that usually enter at certain locations.**

There is a lot about γδ T cells which is still mysterious. For example, it is not known where these cells are educated. Traditional T cells are taught in the thymus not to react against our own self peptides, and although γδ T cells also are found in the thymus, nude mice, which lack a functional thymus, still produce functional γδ T cells. In most cases, it also is not known exactly what the receptors on γδ T cells recognize, but it is believed that, like B cells, γδ T cells focus on unpresented antigen. Finally, the exact mission of γδ T cells is not clear. However, because the receptors of some γδ T cells recognize proteins (e.g., MICA and MICB) which are expressed on the surface of cells that are under stress, it has been postulated that γδ T cells are designed to kill cells that become stressed as the result of a microbial infection.

There is another type of non-traditional T cell that is mentioned frequently, but about which relatively little is known: the NKT cell. In a human, only about 1% of the T cells in the blood are of this type. As its name implies, this non-traditional T cell has some of the properties of the natural killer (NK) cells of the innate system, and some of the properties of traditional T cells of the adaptive immune system. NKT cells mature in the thymus and have αβ receptors. However, in contrast to the αβ receptors of traditional T cells, which are incredibly diverse, the repertoire of receptors expressed by NKT cells is quite limited. In addition, the receptors of NKT cells recognize lipids presented by non-classical, CD1 MHC molecules instead of protein fragments presented by class I or class II MHC molecules.

It has been proposed that NKT cells evolved as a weapon designed to protect us against microbes like tuberculosis which produce characteristic lipid molecules. However, normal mice and mice that have been engineered to lack NKT cells are equally susceptible to infection with TB – so a precise role for NKT cells in protecting us from infection has not been defined.

Because much more is known about traditional T cells than about their non-traditional cousins, and because they seem to be the T cells which are most important for protecting us from disease, we will limit our discussion in this book to T cells of the traditional variety.

HOW A T CELL'S RECEPTORS SIGNAL

Once a TCR has recognized its cognate antigen presented by an MHC molecule, the next step is to transmit a signal from the surface of the T cell, where recognition takes place, to the nucleus of the T cell. The idea is that for the T cell to switch from a resting state to a state of activation, gene expression must be altered, and these genes are, of course, located in the cell's nucleus. Normally, this type of signaling across the cell membrane involves a transmembrane protein that has two parts: an external region which binds to a molecule (called a ligand) that is outside the cell, plus an internal region that initiates a biochemical cascade which conveys the "ligand bound" signal to the nucleus. Here the TCR runs into a bit of a problem. As is true of the BCR, the αβ TCR has a perfectly fine extracellular domain that can bind to its ligand (the combination of MHC molecule and peptide), but the cytoplasmic tails of the α and β proteins are only about three amino acids long – way too short to signal.

To handle the signaling part, Mother Nature had to add a few bells and whistles to the TCR: a complex of proteins collectively called CD3. In humans, this signaling complex is made up of four different proteins: γ, δ, ε, and ζ (gamma, delta, epsilon, and zeta). Please note, however, that the γ and δ proteins that are part of the CD3 complex are not the same as the γ and δ proteins that make up the γδ T cell receptor. The CD3 proteins are anchored in the cell membrane, and have cytoplasmic tails that are long enough to signal just fine.

The whole complex of proteins (α, β, γ, δ, ε, ζ) is transported to the cell surface as a unit. If any one of these proteins fails to be made, you don't get a TCR on the surface. So most immunologists consider the functional, mature TCR to be this whole complex of proteins. After all, the α and β proteins are great for recognition, but they can't signal. And together, the γ, δ, ε, and ζ proteins signal just fine, but they are totally blind to what's going on outside the cell. You need both parts to make it work. As with BCRs, **signaling involves clustering TCRs together in one area of the T cell surface**. When this happens, a threshold number of kinase enzymes is recruited by the cytoplasmic tails of the CD3 proteins, and the activation signal is dispatched to the nucleus.

When the α and β chains of the TCR were first discovered, it was thought that the TCR was just an on/off switch whose only function was to signal activation. But now that you have heard about the CD3 proteins, let me ask you: does this look like a simple on/off switch? No way. Mother Nature certainly wouldn't make an on/off switch with six proteins! No, **this TCR is quite versatile. It can send signals that result in very different outcomes, depending on how, when, and where it is triggered.** For example, when T cells are educated in the thymus, TCRs are used to trigger suicide (death by apoptosis) if the TCR recognizes MHC plus self peptides. Later, if its TCRs recognize their cognate antigen presented by MHC molecules, but a T cell does not receive the required co-stimulatory signals, that T cell may be neutered (anergized) so it can't function. And, of course, when a TCR is presented with its cognate antigen and co-stimulatory signals are available, the TCR signals activation. So this same T cell receptor, depending on the situation, signals death, anergy, or activation. In fact, there are now documented cases in which the alteration of a single amino acid in a presented peptide can change the signal from activation to death! Clearly this is no on/off switch, and immunologists are working very hard to understand exactly how TCR signaling is "wired," and what factors influence the signaling outcome.

CD4 AND CD8 CO-RECEPTORS

In addition to the T cell receptor, there are two more molecules which are involved in antigen recognition by T cells – the CD4 and CD8 co-receptors. Now, doesn't it seem that Mother Nature got carried away when she added on these CD4 and CD8 co-receptors? I mean, there are already two proteins, α and β, to use for antigen recognition, and four more, γ, δ, ε, and ζ, to use for signaling. Wouldn't you think that would do it? Apparently not, so there must be essential features of the system that require CD4 and CD8 co-receptors. Let's see what these might be.

Killer T cells and helper T cells perform two very different functions, and they "look at" two different molecules, class I or class II MHC, respectively, to get their cues. But how do CTLs know to focus on peptides presented by class I molecules – and how do Th cells know to scan APCs for peptides presented by class II? After all, it wouldn't be so great if a CTL got confused, recognized a class II–peptide complex on an APC, and killed the antigen presenting cell! So here's where CD4 and CD8 come in. CTLs generally express CD8 and Th cells usually express CD4. These co-receptor molecules are designed to clip onto either class I MHC (CD8) or class II MHC molecules (CD4).

These "clips" strengthen the adhesion between the T cell and the APC, so **CD4 and CD8 co-receptors function to focus the attention of Th cells and CTLs on the proper MHC molecule.** But there is more to the story, because it turns out that CD4 and CD8 are signaling molecules just like the CD3 complex of proteins. Both CD4 and CD8 have tails that extend through the cell wall and into the interior (cytoplasm) of the cell, and both of these tails have the right characteristics to signal. In addition, because CD4 is a single protein and CD8 is composed of two different proteins, the signals that these co-receptors send are likely to be quite different – perhaps as different as "help" and "kill." In contrast to CD3 molecules, which are glued rather tightly to the αβ T cell receptor on the cell surface, the CD4 and CD8 co-receptors usually are only loosely associated with the TCR/CD3 proteins. The idea is that after a TCR has engaged its cognate antigen presented by an MHC molecule, the CD4 or CD8 co-receptors then clip on and stabilize the TCR-MHC-peptide interaction, thereby strengthening the signal sent by the TCR.

When T cells begin maturing in the thymus, they express both types of co-receptors on their surface. Immunologists call them $CD4^+CD8^+$ cells. Then, as they mature, expression of one or the other of these co-receptors is downregulated, and a cell becomes either $CD4^+$ or $CD8^+$. So how does a given T cell decide whether it will express CD4 or CD8 when it grows up? Well, immunologists are not any more certain about how T cells decide to be $CD4^+$ or $CD8^+$ than they are about how B cells decide to be plasma cells or memory cells. Some think that it is just a random process in which T cells downregulate expression of one type of co-receptor. Others (probably the majority) believe that if a TCR happens to bind, say, to a class I molecule on the surface of a cell in the thymus, a signal is somehow sent to downregulate CD4 expression (the "instructive" model). Although recent experiments favor the instructive model, other experimental results argue against it – so the question of how T cells "pick" their co-receptor molecules is still unanswered.

CO-STIMULATION

In naive T cells, the "connection" between the T cell's receptors and the cell's nucleus is not very good. It's as if the T cell had an electrical system in which a large resistor were placed between the sensor (the TCR) and the piece of equipment it is designed to regulate (gene expression in the nucleus). Because of this "resistor," a lot of the signal from the TCR is lost as it travels to the nucleus. The result is that a prohibitively large number of TCRs would have to engage their cognate antigen before the signal that reaches the nucleus would be strong enough to have any effect. If, however, while the TCRs are engaged, the T cell also receives co-stimulation, the signal from the TCRs is amplified many times, so that fewer (probably about 100-fold fewer) TCRs must be engaged to activate a naive T cell. Although a number of different molecules have been identified which can co-stimulate T cells, cer-

tainly the best studied examples are the B7 proteins (B7-1 and B7-2) which are expressed on the surface of antigen presenting cells. B7 molecules provide co-stimulation to T cells by plugging into receptor molecules called CD28 on the T cell's surface.

So in addition to having their T cell receptors ligated by MHC-peptide, naive T cells must also receive co-stimulatory signals before they can be activated. Co-stimulation can be thought of as an "amplifier" that strengthens the "I'm engaged" signal sent by a T cell's receptors, thereby lowering the threshold number of TCRs which must be crosslinked by MHC–peptide complexes. Interestingly, once a naive T cell has been activated, the connection between the TCRs and the nucleus strengthens. It is as if an experienced T cell has been "rewired" so that the resistor present in a naive T cell is bypassed. As a result of this rewiring, in an experienced T cell, amplification of the TCR signal is not as important as it is in virgin T cells. Consequently, experienced T cells have a reduced requirement for co-stimulation. Recent experiments have suggested a mechanism by which co-stimulation might amplify the TCR signal. Here's how this is thought to work.

Although it is easy to visualize the surface of a cell as a rigid covering, the fact is that the plasma membrane that cloaks a human cell is more like a viscous fluid than a rigid shell. Indeed, proteins that are on the cell surface "float" around fairly freely in this oily gunk. Importantly, the composition of the cell membrane is not homogeneous, and certain proteins and certain types of lipid molecules form aggregates called "rafts." When immunologists examined these cholesterol-rich rafts, they found that they contain a large number of the signaling molecules that are used to carry the "TCR engaged" signal from the cell surface to the nucleus. Immunologists also discovered that before a naive T cell is activated, most of its T cell receptors are not associated with these rafts. However, once a T cell's receptors engage their cognate antigen, the TCRs and the rafts come together. This brings the TCRs into close contact with the downstream signaling molecules, and that completes the circuit to the nucleus.

It turns out that before naive T cells are activated, they don't have many of these lipid rafts on their surface. Most of them are stored inside the cell as parts of other membranous structures. And it is this dearth of rafts on the cell surface that is one of the reasons why the connection between TCRs and the nucleus in a virgin T cell is not a good one – there just aren't enough wires (downstream signaling molecules) available to efficiently carry the signal. However, if a virgin T cell's receptors engage their cognate antigen <u>and</u> appropriate co-stimulation is supplied by the antigen presenting cell, the lipid rafts that are stored inside the cell are rushed to the surface. Now the signal from the TCR can be carried by the additional downstream signaling molecules associated with these rafts, and a strong signal can be sent to the nucleus.

According to this model, the key to signal amplification by co-stimulation is that co-stimulation recruits lipid rafts to the surface of the T cell. Indeed, experienced T cells have many more rafts on their surfaces than do naive cells. This would explain why reactivation of experienced T cells does not require strong co-stimulation – because the rafts in experienced T cells are already on the surface, just waiting to carry the signal.

A TIME-LAPSE PHOTO OF HELPER T CELL ACTIVATION

In the lymph nodes, helper T cells quickly scan dendritic cells to see if their cognate antigen is being displayed. Indeed, a single dendritic cell typically hosts about 1000 such "visits" each hour. If a T cell does find a dendritic cell displaying its cognate antigen, the T cell "lingers," because complete activation of a naive helper T cell actually takes between four and ten hours. During this time, a number of important events take place. First, adhesion molecules on the surface of the dendritic cell bind to their adhesion partners on the T cell, helping keep the two cells together. Next, the CD4 co-receptor molecules on the surface of the T cell clip onto the class II MHC molecules on the dendritic cell and strengthen the interaction between the two cells. In addition, the engagement of its TCRs upregulates the expression of adhesion molecules on the Th cell surface, strengthening the "glue" that holds the APC and the T cell together. This is important, because the binding between a TCR and an MHC–peptide complex is actually rather weak to allow for rapid scanning. Consequently, the Velcro-like adhesion molecules are extremely important for T cell activation. In fact, the ability to express the adhesion molecules required to keep APCs and T cells together long enough for a threshold level of TCR engagement to be reached is one feature that sets APCs apart from "ordinary" cells. The clustering of TCRs and adhesion molecules at the point of contact between an APC and a T cell results in the formation of what immunologists call an "immunological synapse."

Engagement of a helper T cell's receptors also upregulates expression of CD40L proteins on its surface, and when these proteins plug into the CD40 proteins on the surface of a dendritic cell, several remarkable things happen. Although mature dendritic cells express MHC and co-stimulatory molecules (e.g., B7) when they first enter lymph nodes, the expression level of these proteins increases when CD40 proteins on the APC are engaged by the CD40L proteins on a Th cell. In addition, engagement of a dendritic cell's CD40 proteins prolongs the life of the dendritic cell. This extension of a "useful" dendritic cell's life span makes perfect sense. It insures that the particular dendritic cells which are presenting a T cell's cognate antigen will stick around long enough to activate a lot of these T cells. So the interaction between the dendritic cell and a naive helper T cell is not just one way. These cells actually perform an activation "dance" in which they stimulate each other. The end result of this cooperation is that the dendritic cell becomes a more potent antigen presenting cell, and the Th cell is activated to express the high levels of CD40L required for helping activate B cells.

After activation is complete, the helper T cell and the antigen presenting cell part. The APC then goes on to activate other T cells, while the recently activated Th cells proliferate to build up their numbers. During an infection, a single activated T cell can give rise to about 10 000 daughter cells during the first week or so of proliferation. This proliferation is driven by growth factors such as IL-2. Naive T cells can make some IL-2, but they don't have IL-2 receptors on their surface – so they can't respond to this cytokine. In contrast, activated Th cells produce large amounts of IL-2, and they also express receptors for this cytokine on their surface. As a result, newly activated helper T cells stimulate their own proliferation. This coupling of activation to the upregulation of growth factor receptors is the essence of clonal selection: those Th cells which are selected for activation (because their TCRs recognize an invader) upregulate their growth factor receptors, and proliferate to form a clone.

So the sequence of events during the activation of a helper T cell is this. Adhesion molecules mediate weak binding between the Th and the APC while TCRs engage their cognate antigen presented by the APC. Receptor engagement strengthens the adhesion between the two cells, and upregulates CD40L expression on the Th cell. CD40L then binds to CD40 on the APC and stimulates expression of MHC and co-stimulatory molecules on the APC surface. The co-stimulation provided by the APC amplifies the "TCR engaged" signal, making activation of the Th cell more efficient. When activation is complete, the cells disengage, and the Th cell proliferates, driven by growth factors which bind to receptors that appear on the Th cell surface as a result of activation. This proliferation produces a clone of helper T cells which can recognize the invader advertised by the antigen presenting cell.

HOW KILLER T CELLS ARE ACTIVATED

For a helper T cell to be activated, its receptors must recognize their cognate antigen displayed by class II MHC molecules on the surface of an activated dendritic cell, and the Th cell must also receive co-stimulatory signals from that same dendritic cell. This requirement that two cells (the Th cell and the DC) agree that there has been an invasion is a powerful safeguard against the activation of "rogue" helper T cells – cells which might direct an attack against our own tissues, causing autoimmune disease.

Although the events involved in the activation of helper T cells are pretty clear, the picture of how naive killer T cells are activated is still rather fuzzy. Doesn't it seem odd to you that something as important as CTL activation remains rather mysterious? It does to me. However, I think this fact helps explain why immunology is such an interesting subject: There are still many important features of the system to be discovered.

Until recently, it was believed that for a naive killer T cell to be activated, three cells needed to be involved: a CTL with receptors that recognized the invader; an activated dendritic cell, which was using its class I MHC molecules to present the invader's proteins to the CTL; and an activated helper T cell which was providing "help." One way this might happen would be for the dendritic cell, the Th cell, and the CTL to engage in a *ménage à trois*. However, early in an infection, when there are very few of any of these cells around, the probability is quite small that a helper T cell and a killer T cell would simultaneously find a dendritic cell which happens to be presenting their cognate antigen. Moreover, the requirement that three cells (the CTL, the dendritic cell, and the helper T cell) all agree that there is danger seems like overkill in terms of safeguarding against "unauthorized" activation.

Experiments have now shown that, in response to an invasion by microbes which can infect cells (the microbes that CTLs are designed to defend against), T cell help appears not to be required during the initial activation of killer T cells. A two-cell interaction between a naive CTL and an activated dendritic cell is sufficient. During this meeting, the CTL's receptors recognize their cognate antigen displayed by class I MHC molecules on the dendritic cell, and they receive the co-stimulation they need from that same dendritic cell. What this means is that **the way a naive killer T cell is activated is analogous to the way a naive Th cell is activated: by encountering an activated dendritic cell.**

The fact that both helper T cells and CTLs can be activated by a two-cell interaction makes perfect sense in terms of getting the adaptive immune system fired up before invaders take over completely. However, this "helpless" activation of naive killer T cells raises an important question: What then is the role of the "quarterback" Th cell in a CTL's response to an invasion? If Th cells are supposed to be orchestrating the immune response, just what is their contribution in terms of directing killer T cells?

The latest experiments suggest that when CTLs are activated without Th cell help, they proliferate somewhat to build up their numbers and they can kill infected cells. Nevertheless, these helpless T cells do not kill with high efficiency, and they do not live very long. It is as if helpless activation of CTLs results in a small "burst" of killer T cells designed to deal quickly with invaders early in an infection. However, in order to efficiently activate long-lived killer T cells and to generate memory killer T cells – cells which can defend against a subsequent invasion by the same attacker – assistance from helper T cells is required.

It is possible that relatively late in an immune response, there may be enough activated dendritic cells, Th cells, and killer T cells present in lymph nodes and other secondary lymphoid organs to make a three-cell interaction probable. Moreover, there is some evidence that a two-cell meeting between an activated dendritic cell and a helper T cell can generate chemokines which attract killer T cells, making a *ménage à trois* more likely. Recent experiments also suggest that when a helper T cell finds a dendritic cell which is presenting its cognate antigen, these two cells remain "hooked up" for a period of hours – making it more probable that the rare CTL which also recognizes that invader will join the party. Another possibility is that when helper T cells are activated, the dendritic cells which activate them become "licensed" to activate CTLs – thus avoiding the need for all three cells to meet simultaneously.

Although it still isn't clear how Th cell-dependent activation of naive CTLs is accomplished, once CTLs have been activated and have proliferated, they travel to the battle scene. Although a single CTL is capable of killing many target cells sequentially, thousands of cells usually are infected during an attack. So to amplify their killing power, CTLs can proliferate once they reach the battle scene. However, most killer T cells depend on an external supply of the growth factor, IL-2, to proliferate out in the tissues – and helper T cells are the major suppliers of this cytokine. Consequently, **when many CTLs are needed, (e.g., during a viral infection), helper T cells can supply the IL-2 required for killer T cells to proliferate. In this way, helper T cells can control the strength of a killer T cell response.**

THOUGHT QUESTIONS

1. Why do you think six different proteins are required to make up a fully functional T cell receptor?

2. What is the difference between a co-receptor and co-activation? Why is each important?

3. Why are cellular adhesion molecules important during T cell activation? Don't these "sticky" molecules just slow the process down?

4. What safeguards are in place to prevent inappropriate activation of helper and killer T cells?

5. What happens when dendritic cells and helper T cells "dance"?

6. Essentially all players on the innate and adaptive immune system teams must be activated before they can "get into the game." Trace the steps in the "activation cascade" which begins when an LPS-carrying, Gram-negative bacterium enters a wound, and which ends when antibodies are produced that can recognize the bacterium.

7. Why is it that some people seem to have a "good" immune system (i.e., they never get sick), whereas others seem to catch every bug that comes along? Asked another way: Which components of the immune system can differ between individuals?

LECTURE 6

T Cells at Work

REVIEW

I'm sure you have noticed that there are many similarities between the ways B cells and T cells are activated. BCRs and TCRs both have "recognition" proteins that extend outside the cell, and which are incredibly diverse because they are made by a strategy of mixing and matching gene segments. For the BCR, these are the light and heavy chains that make up the antibody molecule. For the TCR, the molecules that recognize antigen are the α and β proteins. TCRs and BCRs have cytoplasmic tails that are too short to signal recognition, so additional molecules are required for this purpose. For the BCR, these signaling proteins are called Igα and Igβ, while for the TCR, signaling involves a complex of proteins called CD3.

For B and T cells to be activated, their receptors must be clustered by antigen, because this crosslinking brings together many of their signaling molecules in a small region of the cell. When the density of signaling molecules is great enough, an enzymatic chain reaction is set off that conveys the "receptor engaged" signal to the cell's nucleus. There, in the "brain center" of the cell, genes involved in activation are turned off or on as a result of this signal.

While crosslinking of receptors is essential for activation, it is not enough. Naive B and T cells also require co-stimulatory signals that are not antigen specific. For B cell activation, a helper T cell can provide co-stimulation through surface proteins called CD40L that plug into CD40 proteins on the B cell surface. For T cells, one form of co-stimulation involves B7 proteins on an activated dendritic cell that engage CD28 proteins on the surface of the T cell.

In addition to recognition and signaling molecules, BCRs and TCRs also associate with co-receptor molecules which serve to amplify the signal that the receptors send. For B

cells, this co-receptor recognizes antigen that has been opsonized by complement. If the BCR recognizes an antigen, and if that antigen also is "decorated" with complement protein fragments, the antigen serves as a "clamp" that brings the BCR and the complement receptor together on the surface of the B cell, greatly amplifying the "receptor engaged" signal. As a consequence, B cells are much more easily activated (many fewer BCRs must be crosslinked) by antigen that has been opsonized by complement.

T cells also have co-receptors. Th cells express CD4 co-receptor molecules on their surface, and CTLs express CD8 co-receptors. When a TCR binds to antigen presented by an MHC molecule, the co-receptor on the T cell surface clips onto the MHC molecule. This serves to strengthen the signal that is sent by the TCR to the nucleus, so that the T cell is more easily activated (fewer TCRs must be crosslinked). These co-receptors only work with the "right" MHC types: class I for CTLs with CD8 co-receptors, and class II for Th cells with CD4 co-receptors. Consequently, co-receptors really are "focus" molecules. The B cell co-receptor helps B cells focus on antigens that have already been identified by the complement system as dangerous (those that have been opsonized). The CD4 co-receptor focuses the attention of Th cells on antigens displayed by class II MHC molecules, and the CD8 co-receptor focuses CTLs on antigens displayed by class I MHC molecules.

Of course, there is an important difference between what B cells and T cells "look at." The BCR recognizes antigen in its "natural" state – that is, antigen which has not been chopped up and bound to MHC molecules. This antigen can be a protein or almost any other organic molecule (e.g., a carbohydrate or a fat). In contrast, the $\alpha\beta$

How the Immune System Works, Fourth Edition. Lauren Sompayrac. © 2012 John Wiley & Sons, Ltd. Published 2012 by John Wiley & Sons, Ltd.

Once helper T cells and killer T cells have been activated, they are ready to go to work – to become, as immunologists say, "effector cells." The primary job of an effector CTL is to kill cells that have been infected by viruses or bacteria. Effector helper T cells have two main duties. First, they can remain in the blood and lymphatic circulation and travel from node to node, providing help for B cells or for killer T cells. The other duty of an effector helper T cell is to exit blood vessels at the sites where a battle is going on to provide help for the soldiers of the innate and adaptive immune systems.

Helper T cells can produce many different cytokines – protein molecules which they use to communicate with the rest of the immune system. As the "quarterback" of the immune system team, the helper T cell uses cytokines to "call the plays." These include cytokines such as TNF, IFN-γ, IL-4, IL-5, IL-6, IL-10, IL-17, and IL-21. However, a single Th cell doesn't secrete all these different cytokines. In fact, Th cells tend to secrete subsets of cytokines – subsets which are appropriate to orchestrate an immune defense against particular invaders. So far, three major subsets have been identified: Th1, Th2, and Th17 (you'll see in a moment why it is Th17 instead of Th3). You shouldn't take this to mean, however, that there are only three different combinations of cytokines that can be secreted by Th cells. In fact, immunologists initially had a hard time finding helper T cells that secreted exactly the Th1 or Th2 cytokine subsets in humans. Clearly, there are helper T cells which secrete mixtures of cytokines that don't conform to the Th1/Th2/Th17 paradigm, but the concept of three major subsets turns out to be quite useful in trying to make sense of the mixture of cytokines (the cytokine "profile") that Th cells produce.

Of course, all of this begs the question: How does a helper T cell know which cytokines are appropriate for a given situation? Well, as any football fan knows, behind every good quarterback there is a good coach.

THE DENDRITIC CELL AS "COACH" OF THE IMMUNE SYSTEM TEAM

For a helper T cell to make an informed decision about which cytokines to make, at least two pieces of information are required. First, it's necessary to know what type of invader the immune system is dealing with. Is it a virus, a bacterium, a parasite, or a fungus? Second, it is essential to determine where in the body the invaders are located. Are they in the respiratory tract, the digestive tract, or the big toe? Virgin helper T cells don't have direct access to either type of information. After all, they are busy circulating through the blood and lymph, trying to find their cognate antigen. What is needed is an "observer" who has actually been at the battle site, who has collected the pertinent information, and who can pass it along to the helper T cell. And which of the immune system cells could qualify as such an observer? The dendritic antigen presenting cell, of course!

Just as the coach of a football team collects information on the opposing team and formulates a game plan, so a dendritic cell, acting as "coach" of the immune system team, collects information on the invasion, and decides how the immune system should react. That's why dendritic cells are so important. They don't just turn naive helper T cells and killer T cells on. They actually function as the "brains" of the immune system, processing the information pertaining to the invasion, and producing a plan of action.

What are the inputs that dendritic cells integrate to produce the game plan? These inputs are of two types. The first input comes to the dendritic cell through its pattern recognition receptors. These are the cellular receptors I mentioned in Lecture 4 which recognize conserved patterns that are characteristic of various classes of invaders. For example, Toll-like receptor 4 (TLR4) senses the presence of LPS, which is a molecule that is a component of the cell walls of Gram-negative bacteria. TLR4 also can detect proteins made by certain viruses. TLR2 specializes in identifying proteins that are "signatures" of Gram-positive bacteria. TLR3 recognizes the double-stranded RNA produced during many viral infections. And TLR9 recognizes the unmethylated DNA di-nucleotide, CpG, which is characteristic of bacterial DNA.

Although TLRs were the first pattern recognition receptors to be characterized, additional families of pattern recognition receptors have now been discovered. Consequently, the emerging picture is that different types of antigen presenting cells (e.g., dendritic cells or macrophages) in different parts of the body display distinct sets of these pattern recognition receptors which are "tuned" to recognize various structural features of common microbial invaders. By integrating the signals from these diverse pattern recognition receptors, an APC gathers information on the type of invader to be defended against.

The second "scouting report" dendritic cells employ when formulating their game plan is received through various cytokine receptors on their surface. Because different pathogens elicit the production of different cytokines during an infection, dendritic cells can learn a lot about an invader by sensing the cytokine environment. Moreover, cells in different areas of the body (e.g., skin cells or cells that underlie the intestines) produce characteristic mixtures of cytokines in response to invaders, and these cytokines help "imprint" dendritic cells with information about the area of the body which is under attack. As a consequence, dendritic cells which observe a battle in one part of the body will have a different character from dendritic cells that are stationed in another area of the body – a "regional identity," if you will.

So **dendritic cells out on the front lines receive input about the invader through pattern recognition receptors and cytokine receptors. It is then up to the dendritic cell to "decode" these inputs and decide what types of weapons need to be mobilized. In addition, the cytokine**

environment in which DCs are activated and the pattern recognition receptors that are triggered imprint DCs with a regional identity. This allows them to remember their "roots" and dispatch the weapons of the adaptive immune system to the region of the body where they are needed.

But how is the dendritic cell's game plan conveyed to the Th cell – the cell that will direct the action? There are two ways that the coach instructs the quarterback. First, there are co-stimulatory molecules which are displayed on the surface of activated dendritic cells, and the particular co-stimulatory molecules that are displayed will depend on the type of invader the dendritic cell has encountered. These surface molecules can "plug into" receptor molecules on the surface of helper T cells to pass this information along. Although B7 is the best-studied co-stimulatory molecule, other co-stimulatory molecules have been identified, and more are certain to be discovered.

In addition to co-stimulatory surface molecules, activated dendritic cells produce cytokines which depend on the identity of the invader, and which can convey information to the helper T cell. So the bottom line is this: **co-stimulatory molecules and cytokines are used by dendritic cells to convey the "game plan" to helper T cells. And the particular combination of co-stimulatory molecules and cytokines which a dendritic cell offers to a Th cell will depend on the scouting report the dendritic cell received at the battle scene.** To get a better idea of how this all works, let's look more closely at the Th1, Th2, and Th17 subsets of cytokines.

Th1 HELPER T CELLS

If you have a puncture wound that results in a bacterial infection or if you are attacked by a virus that replicates in the tissues, resident dendritic cells will be alerted through their pattern recognition receptors and by receiving battle cytokines produced by macrophages and other cells in the inflamed tissues. These signals activate the dendritic cell and imprint it with the special characteristics of a reporter cell which has observed a bacterial or viral infection in the tissues. The details of exactly how this is accomplished aren't clear yet, but the result is that when this DC leaves such a battle site and travels through the lymph to a nearby lymph node, it will produce the cytokine IL-12. And when the IL-12-producing DC presents the battle antigens it has acquired to a virgin helper T cell, that Th cell will be instructed to become a helper T cell which produces the "classical" Th1 cytokines: TNF, IFN-γ, and IL-2.

Why these particular cytokines? Let's see what these cytokines do. The TNF secreted by Th1 helper T cells helps activate macrophages and natural killer cells. However, macrophages only stay activated for a limited time. They are lazy fellows which like to go back to "resting and garbage collecting." Fortunately, the IFN-γ produced by Th1 cells acts as a "prod" that keeps macrophages fired up and engaged in the battle. IFN-γ also influences B cells during class switching to produce human IgG3 antibodies. These antibodies are especially good at opsonizing viruses and bacteria and at fixing complement.

NK cells can kill three or four target cells in about 16 hours, but then they "tire out." The IL-2 produced by Th1 cells can "recharge" NK cells, enabling them to kill some more. In addition, IL-2 is a growth factor which stimulates the proliferation of CTLs, NK cells, and Th1 cells themselves, so that more of these important weapons will be available to deal with the attack.

Altogether, the Th1 cytokines are the perfect package to help defend against a viral or bacterial attack in the tissues. The Th1 cytokines instruct the innate and adaptive systems to produce cells and antibodies that are especially effective against these invaders, and keep the warriors of the immune system fired up until the invaders have been defeated.

Th2 HELPER T CELLS

Now suppose that you have been infected by a parasite (e.g., hookworms) or you have eaten some food that is contaminated with pathogenic bacteria. In the tissues that line your intestines, a battle will be raging. Dendritic cells

from that area will travel to nearby lymph nodes, and will activate those helper T cells which have T cell receptors that can recognize the worm or bacterial antigens presented by the DC. This interaction results in helper T cells which are "programmed" to produce the Th2 subset of cytokines, which includes IL-4, IL-5, and IL-13.

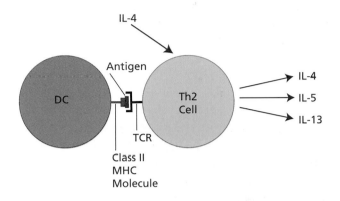

Why IL-4, IL-5, and IL-13, you ask? IL-4 is a growth factor that stimulates the proliferation of helper T cells which have committed to secrete the Th2 profile of cytokines. So, like Th1 cells, Th2 cells produce their own growth factor. IL-4 also is a growth factor for B cells, and this cytokine can influence B cells to class switch to produce IgE antibodies – powerful weapons against parasites such as hookworms. IL-5 is a cytokine which encourages B cells to produce IgA antibodies, antibodies that are especially useful against bacteria which invade via the digestive tract. And IL-13 stimulates the production of mucus in the intestines, which helps prevent more intestinal parasites or pathogenic bacteria from breaching the intestinal wall and entering the tissues. So the Th2 cytokine profile is just the ticket if you need to defend against parasites or pathogenic bacteria that have invaded via the digestive tract.

Now I want to call your attention to two interesting points. First, in the figure above, you will notice that IL-4, which causes a naive Th cell to commit to becoming a Th2 cell, does not come from the dendritic cell. In fact, the source of IL-4 which initiates the Th2 commitment is still a mystery. Of course, once the helper T cell commits to the Th2 cytokine profile, there will be plenty of IL-4 around – because this is one of the cytokines Th2 cells secrete. However, the initial source of IL-4 required for Th2 commitment has not yet been identified.

The second interesting point is that Th2 cells produce cytokines (IL-4 and IL-5) which can influence B cells to make either IgE antibodies (to defend against parasites) or IgA antibodies (to defend against pathogenic bacteria). However, it would be unusual for a person to be infected with parasites and pathogenic bacteria simultaneously. Consequently, you wouldn't want Th2 cells to influence B cells to make both IgE and IgA antibodies. That would be wasteful (and probably dangerous). So how does a Th2 cell decide whether to instruct B cells to make IgE or IgA antibodies?

Immunologist don't have a complete answer to this question, but a major factor in this decision is the location from which the dendritic cells are dispatched. I mentioned earlier that DCs have a "regional identity." For example, there are dendritic cells which reside in "Peyer's patches" – special areas of the intestine that are important in defending against pathogenic bacteria which have been ingested. These particular dendritic cells are "imprinted" by the environment of the Peyer's patch to deliver signals (e.g., via co-stimulatory molecules) to Th cells which cause them to assist with IgA antibody production. On the other hand, dendritic cells which are stationed beneath areas of the intestine that are susceptible to invasion by parasites are imprinted so that they convey signals to Th cells which bias them to help B cells produce IgE antibodies. That's the basic idea, but the details have yet to be worked out.

Th17 HELPER T CELLS

The existence of helper T cells which produce the Th17 cytokine profile is a recent discovery, and less is known about Th17 cells than about Th1 and Th2 helper T cells. One reason for this is that Th17 cells function, at least in part, in the defense against fungi – and the immune system's response to a fungal attack is not nearly so well researched as the immune defense against bacteria and viruses. Consequently, the story on Th17 cells is far from complete, but here is the emerging picture.

If a dendritic cell is stationed in an area of the body which is being attacked by fungi (e.g., a vaginal yeast infection) or certain extracellular bacteria, that DC will travel to a nearby lymph node and activate those helper T cells which recognize the antigens the DC is presenting. These traveling dendritic cells will produce TGFβ and IL-6, which together with co-stimulatory molecules, influence newly activated helper T cells to produce the Th17 subset of cytokines, which includes IL-17 and IL-21.

IL-21 is a growth factor for Th17 cells, so once these helper T cells have committed to being Th17 cells, they stimulate themselves and other Th17 cells to proliferate. This increases the number of cells which can battle the fungus. Secretion of the "signature cytokine," IL-17, results in the recruitment of massive numbers of neutrophils to the site of infection. These neutrophils help defend against pathogens against which Th1 and Th2 cells are relatively ineffective, including fungi and some extracellular bacteria – bacteria which do not enter cells. Indeed, patients who have a genetic defect in IL-17 secretion suffer from devastating fungal infections (e.g., infection with the common yeast, *Candida albicans*) even though their Th1 and Th2 helper T cells function normally. Finally, IL-17 and IL-21 influence B cells to produce antibody classes which can opsonize fungi or bacteria and can activate the complement system. **So if you are attacked by fungi or extracellular bacteria, the cytokines secreted by Th17 cells are there to help protect you.**

Th0 HELPER T CELLS

Some helper T cells (the so-called "Th0" cells) remain "unbiased" when they first are activated, retaining the ability to produce a wide range of cytokines. It appears that DCs tell these helper T cells where to go, but not what to do. However, once Th0 cells reach the battle scene, the cytokine environment they encounter there causes them to commit to the cytokine profile required for the defense. For example, when Th0 cells exit the blood to fight a bacterial infection in the tissues, they encounter an environment rich in IL-12. This is because Th1 cells that are already fighting the bacteria there produce IFN-γ. This cytokine, together with danger signals like the bacterial molecule LPS, activates tissue macrophages, which secrete large amounts of IL-12. And when Th0 cells receive the IL-12 signal, they "realize" what type of battle is being fought, and commit to becoming Th1 cells – which produce the cytokines needed to defend against the bacteria.

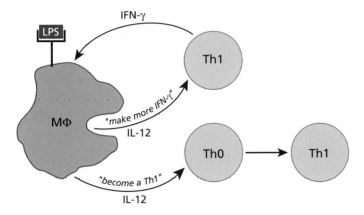

Likewise, Th0 cells can become Th2 or Th17 cells when they reach a battle site that is rich in IL-4 or IL-6 and TGFβ, respectively. So **previously uncommitted Th0 cells can be "converted" by the cytokine environment at the scene of the battle to become Th1, Th2, or Th17 cells.**

LOCKING IN THE HELPER T CELL PROFILE

Once helper T cells commit to producing a particular cytokine profile, they begin to secrete growth factors which are specific for that particular type of Th cell – be it Th1, Th2, or Th17. This sets up a positive feedback loop in which the "selected" Th cell proliferates and produces even more of its own growth factor – triggering further proliferation of this type of helper T cell.

In addition to positive feedback, there is also negative feedback at work. For example, IFN-γ made by Th1 cells actually decreases the rate of proliferation of Th2 cells, so that fewer Th2 cells will be produced. And one of the Th2 cytokines, IL-10, acts to decrease the rate of proliferation of Th1 cells. **The result of all this positive and negative feedback is a large number of helper T cells which are strongly biased toward the production of a certain subset of cytokines.** However, there is one important point which I want to be sure that you understand. **Cytokines have a very limited range. They can travel only short distances in the body before they are captured** by cellular receptors or are degraded. Consequently, **when we talk about helper T cells being biased toward secreting a certain cytokine profile, we are talking about something very local.** Clearly, you wouldn't want every Th cell in your body to be of the Th1 type, because then you'd have no way to defend against a respiratory infection. Conversely, you wouldn't want to have only Th2 cells, because the IgA or IgE antibodies made in response to the Th2 cytokines would be useless if you get a bacterial infection in your big toe. In fact, **it is the local nature of cytokine signaling which gives the immune system the flexibility to simultaneously mount defenses against many different invaders that threaten different parts of the body.**

It is also important to note that dendritic cells are members of the innate system team. Consequently, **the innate immune system not only informs the adaptive system when there is danger, but the innate system also "coaches" the adaptive system to insure that the appropriate weapons are sent to the right places.**

SUMMARY

To summarize, dendritic cells are stationed beneath all exposed surfaces, where they wait for information on the identity of invaders which breach the barrier defenses. This information is collected by receptors that recognize either molecular patterns that are characteristic of classes of invaders, or cytokines produced by other cells in response to the invasion. Dendritic cells then integrate all this information, and travel to nearby lymph nodes. There they use various combinations of co-stimulatory molecules and cytokines to tell helper T cells where the battle is being fought, and to influence these helper T cells to commit to the production of those cytokines which will orchestrate an immune response appropriate for the particular invader.

Once a Th cell has committed to produce a particular cytokine profile, it begins to secrete growth factors which stimulate the proliferation of that particular Th subset: Th1 cells secrete IFN-γ, Th2 cells secrete IL-4, and Th17 cells secrete IL-21. These committed T cells then either circulate in the blood/lymphatic system to provide help (and instruction) for B cells, or exit the blood at sites of infection to join the battle. Other, uncommitted Th0 cells are dispatched to the battle scene where, under the influence of the battle cytokines, they too become committed to secreting a particular cytokine profile. And once a Th cytokine profile has been established, positive and negative feedback tend to lock in this particular profile.

DELAYED TYPE HYPERSENSITIVITY

There is an example of "signal calling" by Th cells that I think you'll find interesting. It is termed "delayed type hypersensitivity" (DTH), and it was first observed by Robert Koch when he was studying tuberculosis back in the latter part of the nineteenth century. Koch purified a protein, tuberculin, from the bacterium that causes tuberculosis, and used this protein to devise his famous "tuberculin skin test." If you've had this test, you'll recall that a nurse injected something under your skin, and told you to check that area in a few days. If the spot where you were injected became red and swollen, you were instructed to come back in to see the doctor. Here's what that's all about.

The "something" you were injected with was Koch's tuberculin protein. If you have active TB or have been infected with it in the past, your immune system will include memory, Th1-type helper T cells which were made in response to the infection. These experienced cells can recognize the tuberculin fragments presented by dendritic cells stationed beneath the skin and be reactivated. Now the fun begins, because these Th cells secrete IFN-γ and TNF – Th1-type cytokines that activate resident tissue macrophages near the site of injection, and help recruit neutrophils and additional macrophages to the area. The result is a local inflammatory reaction with redness and swelling: the signal that your TB test is positive. Of course, the reason you have to wait several days for the test to "develop" is that memory helper T cells must be reactivated, proliferate, and produce those all-important cytokines that orchestrate the inflammatory reaction. On the other hand, if you have never been exposed to the tuberculosis bacterium, you will have no memory helper T cells to reactivate. Without the cytokines supplied by activated Th cells, there will be no inflammatory reaction to the tuberculin protein, and your skin test will be scored as negative.

What is interesting here is that **delayed type hypersensitivity is both specific and non-specific. The specificity comes from Th cells that direct the immune response after recognizing the tuberculin peptide presented by dendritic cells. The non-specific part of the reaction involves the neutrophils and macrophages that are** recruited and activated by cytokines secreted by the Th cells. This is yet another example of the cooperation that goes on between the adaptive and innate immune systems.

You may be wondering why the tuberculin used for the test doesn't activate naive T cells, so that the next time you are tested, you will get a positive reaction. The reason is that the tuberculin protein does not, by itself, cause an inflammatory reaction (i.e., a battle situation), and you remember that dendritic cells only mature and carry antigen to a lymph node if a battle is on. So if a protein is injected under your skin and it does not cause inflammation (i.e., it is ignored by the innate system), the adaptive immune system will not be activated. This illustrates again how important the innate immune system is for initiating an immune response: **if your innate system does not recognize an invader as dangerous and put up a fight, your adaptive system usually will just ignore the invasion.**

HOW CTLs KILL

So far in this lecture, we have discussed what activated helper T cells do. Now it is time to focus on killer T cells. Once a CTL has been activated, it proliferates rapidly to build up its numbers. These effector T cells then leave the lymph node, enter the blood, and travel to the area of the body where the invaders they can kill are located. When an effector T cells reaches the battle site, it exits the blood, and begins to hack away at infected cells. Most killing by CTLs requires contact between the CTL and its target cell, and CTLs have several weapons they can use during this "hand-to-hand" combat.

One weapon CTLs employ involves the production of a protein called perforin. Perforin is a close relative of the C9 complement protein that is part of the membrane attack complex, and, like its cousin, perforin can bind to cell membranes and drill holes in them. Two theories have been advanced to try to explain how a CTL uses perforin to kill. In both, a killer T cell's TCRs first identify the target. Then adhesion molecules on the CTL hold the target cell close while the killer cell delivers a mixture of perforin and an enzyme called granzyme B onto the surface of the target cell. According to the first theory, perforin then makes a hole in the cell's outer membrane and granzyme B is delivered through this hole into the cytoplasm of the cell. The second theory holds that the target cell encloses both granzyme B and perforin in a pouch (vesicle) made from the target cell's membrane. Once inside the target cell, the perforin molecules then make holes in this vesicle, allowing the granzyme B to escape into the cytoplasm of the cell. After a killer T cell has made contact with its target, it only takes about half an hour to kill the cell, and during each attack, the CTL only uses a fraction of its perforin and granzyme B. Consequently, a single killer T cell can execute multiple target cells.

Although the mechanism of action is not well understood, the bottom line is that **perforin somehow helps a CTL deliver granzyme B into the cytoplasm of its target cell. There, granzyme B triggers an enzymatic chain reaction which causes the cell to commit suicide by apoptosis.** This kind of "assisted suicide" usually involves the self-destruction of the target cell's DNA by its own enzymes. An important feature of this type of killing is that it is "directed." The CTL delivers its lethal cargo right onto the target cell, so that other cells in the area are not damaged during the slaughter.

The second way a CTL can kill is by using a protein on its surface called Fas ligand (FasL) which can bind to (ligate) the Fas protein on the surface of a target cell. When this happens, a suicide program is set in motion within the target cell, and, again, the cell dies by apoptosis. Interestingly, natural killer cells use these same two mechanisms (perforin/granzyme B and FasL) to kill their targets.

It is worth mentioning here that **there actually are two different ways a cell can die: by necrosis or by apoptosis.** Although the end result is the same (a dead cell), the two processes are quite different. Cells usually die by necrosis either as the result of a wound (e.g., a cut or a burn) or when they are killed by an attacking virus or bacterium. **During necrosis, enzymes and chemicals that normally are safely contained within a living cell are released by the dying cell into the surrounding tissues, where they can do real damage.** In contrast, death by apoptosis is much tidier. As a cell dies by apoptosis, its contents are enclosed in vesicles made from the outer membrane of the dying cell. These vesicles are then eaten and destroyed by nearby macrophages as part of their garbage collecting duty. Consequently, **during apoptosis, the contents of the target cell don't get out into the tissues to cause damage.** So by killing their targets by inducing apoptosis rather than necrosis, CTLs can rid the body of virus-infected cells without causing the collateral tissue damage that would result from necrotic cell death.

There is another reason why triggering cells to die by apoptosis is an especially effective way for killer T cells to destroy virus-infected cells. **When virus-infected cells die by apoptosis, the DNA of unassembled viruses is destroyed along with the target cell's DNA. In addition, DNA or RNA viruses that have reached various stages of assembly within the cell are enclosed in apoptotic vesicles and are disposed of by macrophages. It is this ability to kill infected cells and the viruses they contain by inducing apoptosis that makes a killer T cell such a potent, anti-viral weapon.**

EPILOGUE

You should now be familiar with all of the major players of the innate and adaptive immune systems. For this defense to function properly, however, the movements of the various players must be carefully choreographed to enhance cooperation – and to make sure that the appropriate weapons are delivered to the locations within the body where they are needed. How all this is accomplished is the subject of our next lecture.

SUMMARY FIGURE

Here is our final summary figure, showing both the innate and adaptive systems – and the network they form. Can you identify all the players, and do you understand how they interact with each other?

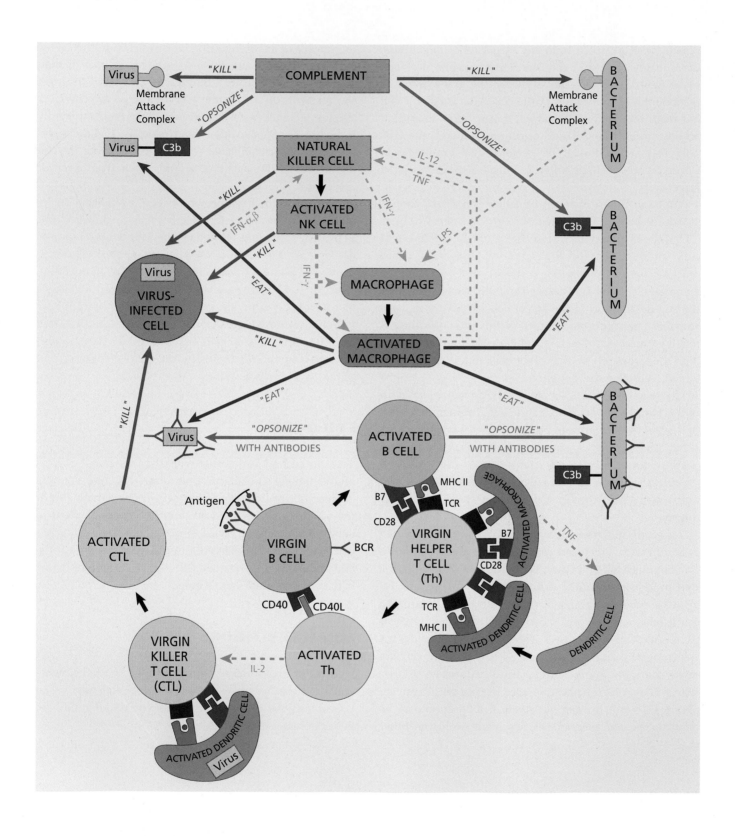

THOUGHT QUESTIONS

1. How does a helper T cell know which cytokine profile to produce?

2. How does a helper T cell "call the plays" for B cells?

3. How does a helper T cell "call the plays" for killer T cells?

4. How does a helper T cell orchestrate the actions of innate system players like macrophages and NK cells?

5. Why is it advantageous to have Th0 helper T cells, which don't commit to a particular cytokine profile until they reach the battle scene?

6. Cytokines have a limited range. Why is this a good thing?

LECTURE 7

Secondary Lymphoid Organs and Lymphocyte Trafficking

REVIEW

Certainly one of the most elegant features of the immune system is the way Mother Nature arranges to "let the punishment fit the crime," so that exactly the right weapons are mobilized to defend against particular invaders. In your body, dendritic antigen presenting cells are stationed beneath all surfaces that are exposed to the outside world. By virtue of this geographic location, they can observe an invasion firsthand. In fact, the intelligence they acquire at the scene of the battle is complete enough to allow them to formulate a game plan for the rest of the immune system. This information is gathered in part through the dendritic cell's pattern recognition receptors, which detect "signatures" common to different types of invaders. Dendritic cells also have receptors which sense the cytokines given off by other immune system cells that are engaged in the battle. In addition, cells which reside in different areas of the body give off cytokines that imprint the dendritic cell with a regional identity – so it "remembers" where the battle is taking place.

Armed with all this information on the type of invader and the location of the attack, dendritic cells travel to nearby lymph nodes, where they activate T cells. During this process, the game plan is conveyed to helper T cells in the form of co-stimulatory molecules and cytokines expressed by the dendritic cells. This information instructs helper T cells which cytokines to make to orchestrate the appropriate defense against a particular invader. In a sense, the dendritic cell functions as the "coach" of the immune system team, while the Th cell performs the duties of "quarterback," calling the plays designed by the coach. The dendritic cell is part of the innate immune system. Consequently, the innate system not only determines when the adaptive system should be activated in response to danger, but it also instructs the adaptive system on which weapons to deploy and where to send them.

In response to the instructions delivered by dendritic cells, helper T cells produce combinations of cytokines that mobilize the weapons which are especially suited to deal with the invader that is attacking at the moment. Although there are many different cytokines which a given Th cell can secrete, the best studied combinations are called Th1, Th2, and Th17. Th1 cytokines are especially good at organizing the immune defense against viruses and bacteria which infect human cells. Th2 helper T cells produce a combination of cytokines that is just right for defending against parasites or against bacteria that have breached the intestinal barrier. And Th17 helper T cells secrete cytokines that mobilize the immune system to defend against fungi or extracellular bacteria. All of the cytokines produced by helper T cells have a very short range, so their effects are quite "local." This feature allows the immune system to defend against different types of invaders which attack different parts of the body.

When we are attacked by viruses or bacteria which infect human cells, dendritic cells activate killer T cells, and dispatch them to the area of the body which is under attack. Killer T cells destroy infected cells by forcing them to commit suicide – a process called apoptosis. And when the cell dies, the infecting pathogen dies with it.

Up to this point, we've discussed the various elements of innate and adaptive immunity, and how they interact to make an integrated defense system. However, to really understand how this system works, one must have a clear picture of where in the body all these interactions take place. So in this lecture, we're going to focus on the "geography"of the immune system.

The immune system's defense against an attacker actually has three phases: recognition of danger, production of weapons appropriate for the invader, and transport of these weapons to the site of attack. The recognition phase of the adaptive immune response takes place in the "secondary lymphoid organs." These include the lymph nodes, the spleen, and the mucosal-associated lymphoid tissue (called the MALT for short). You may be wondering: if these are the secondary lymphoid organs, what are the primary ones? **The primary lymphoid organs are the bone marrow, where B and T cells are born, and the thymus, where T cells receive their early training.**

LYMPHOID FOLLICLES

All secondary lymphoid organs have one anatomical feature in common: they all contain lymphoid follicles. These follicles are critical for the functioning of the adaptive immune system, so we need to spend a little time getting familiar with them. Lymphoid follicles start life as "primary" lymphoid follicles: loose networks of follicular dendritic cells (FDCs) embedded in regions of the secondary lymphoid organs that are rich in B cells. So **lymphoid follicles are really islands of follicular dendritic cells within a sea of B cells.**

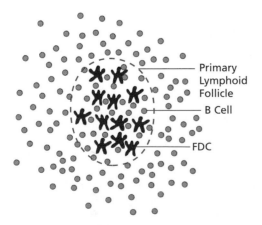

Primary Lymphoid Follicle

B Cell

FDC

Although FDCs also have a starfish-like shape, they are very different from the antigen presenting dendritic cells

(DCs) we talked about before. Those dendritic cells are white blood cells that are produced in the bone marrow, and which then migrate to their sentinel positions in the tissues. In contrast, follicular dendritic cells are regular old cells (like skin cells or liver cells) that take up their final positions in the secondary lymphoid organs as the embryo develops. In fact, follicular dendritic cells are already in place during the second trimester of gestation. Not only are the origins of follicular dendritic cells and antigen presenting dendritic cells quite different, these two types of starfish-shaped cells have very different functions. **Whereas the role of dendritic APCs is to present antigen to T cells via MHC molecules, the function of follicular dendritic cells is to display antigen to B cells.** Here's how this works.

Early in an infection, complement proteins bind to invaders, and some of this complement-opsonized antigen will be delivered by the lymph or blood to the secondary lymphoid organs. Follicular dendritic cells that reside in these organs have receptors on their surface which bind complement fragments, and as a result, follicular dendritic cells pick up and retain the opsonized antigen. In this way, **follicular dendritic cells become "decorated" with antigens that are derived from the battle which is being waged out in the tissues. Moreover, by capturing large numbers of antigens and by holding them close together, FDCs display antigens in a way that can crosslink B cell receptors.** Later during the battle, when antibodies have been produced, **invaders opsonized by antibodies also can be retained on the surface of follicular dendritic cells, because FDCs have receptors that can bind to the constant regions of antibody molecules.**

So follicular dendritic cells capture opsonized antigens and "advertise" these antigens to B cells in a configuration that can help activate them. Those B cells whose receptors are crosslinked by their cognate antigens hanging from these follicular dendritic "trees" proliferate to build up their numbers. And once this happens, the "follicle" begins to grow and become a center of B cell development. Such an active lymphoid follicle is called a "secondary" lymphoid follicle or a "germinal center." The role of complement-opsonized antigen in triggering the development of a germinal center cannot be overemphasized: lymphoid follicles in humans who have a defective complement system never progress past the primary stage. Thus, we see again that **for the adaptive immune system to respond, the innate system must first react to impending danger.**

As B cells proliferate in germinal centers, they become very "fragile." Unless they receive the proper "rescue" signals, they will commit suicide (die by apoptosis). Fortunately, helper T cells that have been activated in the T cell areas of the secondary lymphoid organs migrate to the lymphoid follicle to rescue these B cells. Activated Th cells express high levels of CD40L proteins that can plug into CD40 proteins on the surface of the B cell. When a B cell whose receptors are crosslinked by antigen receives this co-stimulatory signal, it is temporarily rescued from apoptotic death, and continues to proliferate.

The rate at which B cells multiply in a germinal center is truly amazing – the number of B cells can double every six hours! These proliferating B cells push aside other B cells that have not been activated, and establish a region of the germinal center called the "dark zone" – because it contains so many proliferating B cells that it looks dark under a microscope.

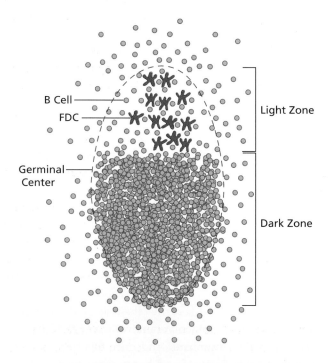

After this period of proliferation, some of the B cells "choose" to become plasma B cells and leave the germinal center. Others, during their time of proliferation, undergo somatic hypermutation to fine tune their receptors. After each round of mutation, the affinity of the mutated BCR is tested. Those B cells whose mutated BCRs do not have a high enough affinity for antigen will die by apoptosis, and will be eaten by macrophages in the germinal center. In contrast, B cells are rescued from apoptosis if the affin-

ity of their receptors is great enough to be efficiently crosslinked by their cognate antigen displayed on FDCs – and if they also receive co-stimulation from activated Th cells that are present in the light zone of the germinal center. The current picture is that B cells "cycle" between periods of proliferation and mutation in the dark zone and periods of testing and restimulation in the light zone. Sometime during all this action, probably in the dark zone, B cells can switch the class of antibody they produce.

In summary, lymphoid follicles are specialized regions of secondary lymphoid organs in which B cells percolate through a lattice of follicular dendritic cells that have captured opsonized antigen on their surface. B cells that encounter their cognate antigen and receive T cell help are rescued from death. These "saved" B cells proliferate and can undergo somatic hypermutation and class switching. Clearly lymphoid follicles are extremely important for B cell development. That's why all secondary lymphoid organs have them.

HIGH ENDOTHELIAL VENULES

A second anatomical feature common to all secondary lymphoid organs except the spleen is the "high endothelial venule" (HEV). **The reason HEVs are so important is that they are the "doorways" through which B and T cells enter these secondary lymphoid organs from the blood.** Most endothelial cells that line the inside of blood vessels resemble overlapping shingles which are tightly "glued" to the cells adjacent to them to prevent the loss of blood cells into the tissues. In contrast, the small blood vessels that collect blood from the capillary beds (the postcapillary venules) within most secondary lymphoid organs are lined with special endothelial cells that are shaped more like a column than like a shingle.

These tall cells are the high endothelial cells. So a high endothelial venule is a special region in a small blood vessel (venule) where there are high endothelial cells. Instead of being glued together, high endothelial cells are "spot welded." As a result, there is enough space between the cells of the HEV for lymphocytes to wriggle through. Actually, "wriggle" may not be quite the right term, because lymphocytes exit the blood very efficiently at these high endothelial venules: about 10 000 lymphocytes exit the blood and enter an average lymph node each second by passing between high endothelial cells.

A TOUR OF THE SECONDARY LYMPHOID ORGANS

Now that you are familiar with lymphoid follicles and high endothelial venules, we are ready to take a tour of some of the secondary lymphoid organs. On our tour today, we will visit a lymph node, a Peyer's patch (an example of the MALT), and the spleen. As we explore these organs, you will want to pay special attention to the "plumbing." How an organ is connected to the blood and lymphatic systems gives important clues about how it functions.

Lymph node architecture
A lymph node is a plumber's dream. This organ has incoming lymphatics which bring lymph into the node, and outgoing lymphatics through which lymph exits. In addition, there are small arteries (arterioles) that carry the blood that nourishes the cells of the lymph node, and veins through which this blood leaves the node. If you look carefully at this figure, you also can see the high endothelial venules.

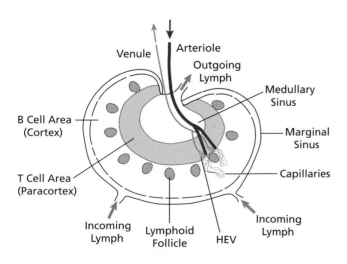

With this diagram in mind, can you see how lymphocytes (B and T cells) enter a lymph node? That's right, they can enter from the blood by pushing their way between the cells of the high endothelial venules. There is also another way lymphocytes can enter the lymph node: with the lymph. After all, lymph nodes are like "dating bars," positioned along the route the lymph takes on its way to be reunited with the blood – and B and T cells actively engage in "bar hopping," being carried from node to node by the lymph. Although lymphocytes have two ways to gain entry to a lymph node, they only exit via the lymph – those high endothelial venules won't let them back into the blood.

Since lymph nodes are places where lymphocytes find their cognate antigen, we also need to discuss how this antigen gets there. When dendritic cells stationed out in the tissues are stimulated by battle signals, they leave the tissues via the lymph, and carry the antigen they have acquired at the battle scene into the secondary lymphoid organs. So this is one way antigen can enter a lymph node: as "cargo" aboard an APC. In addition, antigen which has been opsonized, either by complement or by antibodies, can be carried by the lymph into the node. There the opsonized antigen will be captured by follicular dendritic cells for display to B cells.

When lymph enters a node, it percolates through holes in the marginal sinus (sinus is a fancy word for "cavity"), through the cortex and paracortex, and finally into the medullary sinus – from whence it exits the node via the outgoing lymphatic vessels.

One of the functions of a lymph node is as a "lymph filter." The walls of the marginal sinus are lined with macrophages which capture and devour pathogens as they enter a lymph node. This substantially reduces the number of invaders that the adaptive immune system will need to deal with.

Lymph nodes are centers of activation
The high endothelial venules are located in the paracortex, so lymphocytes pass through this region of the node when they arrive from the blood. In fact, T cells tend to accumulate in the paracortex, being retained there by adhesion molecules. This accumulation of T cells makes good sense, because dendritic cells also are found in the paracortex – and of course, one object of this game is to get T cells together with these antigen presenting cells.

As a helper T cell passes through the paracortex of a lymph node, there is a chance it will encounter a dendritic cell that is presenting its cognate antigen. If so, the Th cell will be activated and will begin to proliferate. This proliferation phase lasts a few days. Most of these newly activated Th cells will then exit the node via the lymph, recirculate through the blood, and re-enter lymph nodes via high endothelial venules. This process of recirculation is fast – it generally takes less than a day – and it is extremely important. Here's why.

There are four major ingredients which must be "mixed" before the adaptive immune system can produce antibodies: APCs to present antigen to Th cells, Th cells with receptors that recognize the presented antigen, opsonized antigen displayed by follicular dendritic cells, and B cells with receptors that recognize the antigen. Early in an infection, there are very few of these ingredients around, and naive B and T cells just circulate through the secondary lymphoid organs at random, checking for a match to their receptors. So the probability is pretty small that the rare Th cell which recognizes a particular antigen will arrive at the very same lymph node that is being visited by the rare B cell with specificity for that same antigen. However, if activated Th cells first proliferate to build up their numbers, and then recirculate to lots of lymph nodes and other secondary lymphoid organs, the Th cells with the right stuff get "spread around," so they have a much better chance of encountering those rare B cells which require their help.

If recirculating Th cells enter a node where their cognate antigen is being presented, they will be restimulated. Some of the restimulated Th cells will proliferate more and recirculate again to spread the help even further. Other restimulated Th cells will move to the lymphoid follicles of a lymph node to provide help to needy B cells, and still others will exit the blood to provide cytokine help to warriors doing battle in the tissues.

Killer T cells also are activated in the paracortex of the lymph node if they find their cognate antigen presented there by dendritic cells. Once activated, CTLs proliferate and recirculate. Some of these CTLs re-enter secondary lymphoid organs and begin this cycle again, whereas others exit the blood at sites of infection to kill pathogen-infected cells.

B cells also engage in cycles of activation, proliferation, circulation, and restimulation. B cells which have encountered their cognate antigen displayed on follicular dendritic cells migrate to the border of the lymphoid follicle where they meet activated T cells that have migrated there from the paracortex. It is during this meeting that B cells first receive the co-stimulation they require for acti-

vation. Both B and T cells then enter the lymphoid follicles, and the B cells proliferate. Many of the newly made B cells exit the lymphoid follicle via the lymph. Some become plasma cells that take up residence in the spleen or bone marrow where they pump out antibodies. Others recirculate through the lymph and blood, and re-enter secondary lymphoid organs. As a result, activated B cells are spread around to secondary lymphoid organs where, if they are restimulated in lymphoid follicles, they can proliferate more and can undergo somatic hypermutation and class switching.

The frantic activity in germinal centers generally is over in about three weeks. By this time, the invader usually has been repulsed, and a lot of the opsonized antigen has been "picked" from the follicular dendritic trees by B cells. At this point, most B cells will have left the follicles or will have died there, and the areas that once were germinal centers will look much more like primary lymphoid follicles.

Lymph node choreography

From this discussion, it should be clear that **a lymph node is a highly organized place with specific areas for antigen presenting cells, T lymphocytes, and B lymphocytes.** But how do APCs and lymphocytes know where to go within a lymph node and when to go there? It turns out that the movements of these cells in this secondary lymphoid organ are carefully controlled using special cytokines called "chemokines" (short for chemoattractive cytokines). Here's how this works.

Follicular dendritic cells in a lymph node produce a chemokine called CXCL13. Naive B cells which enter the node express receptors for this chemokine, and are attracted to the area of the node where the FDCs are displaying opsonized antigen. If a B cell finds its cognate antigen advertised there, it downregulates expression of the receptors for CXCL13, and upregulates expression of another chemokine receptor, CCR7. This receptor detects a chemokine that is produced by cells in the region of the lymph node where activated Th cells and B cells meet – the border between the B and T cell areas. Consequently, once a B cell has found its antigen, it is attracted by the "smell" of this chemokine to the correct location to receive help from activated Th cells.

Likewise, Th cells which have been activated by dendritic cells in the T cell areas of the node also upregulate expression of receptors which cause them to be attracted to the border of the follicle, where B cells that have found their cognate antigen are waiting for T cell help. Then, at a later time, some of these Th cells lose the CCR7 "border" receptor and upregulate a receptor which guides them into the B cell follicles – where they provide help for class switching and somatic hypermutation. So **the movement of immune system cells through a lymph node is orchestrated by the up- and down-regulation of chemokine receptors, and the localized production of chemokines that can be detected by these receptors.**

Now, of course, human cells don't come equipped with little propellers like some bacteria do, so they can't "swim" in the direction of the source of a chemokine. What human cells do is "crawl." In general terms, the end of the cell that senses the greatest concentration of the chemokine "reaches out" toward the chemokine source, and the other end of the cell is retracted. By repeating this motion, a cell can crawl toward the source of a cytokine.

In summary, **lymph nodes act as "lymph filters" which intercept antigen that arrives from infected tissues either alone or as dendritic cell cargo. These nodes provide a concentrated and organized environment of antigen, APCs, T cells, and B cells in which naive B and T cells can be activated, and experienced B and T cells can be restimulated. In a lymph node, naive B and T cells can mature into effector cells that produce antibodies (B cells), provide cytokine help (Th cells), and kill infected cells (CTLs). In short, a lymph node can do it all.**

As everyone knows, lymph nodes that drain sites of infection tend to swell. For example, if you have a viral infection of your upper respiratory tract (e.g., influenza), the cervical nodes in your neck may become swollen. This swelling is due in part to the proliferation of lymphocytes within the node. In addition, cytokines produced by helper T cells in an active lymph node recruit additional macrophages which tend to plug up the medullary sinus. As a result, fluid is retained in the node, causing further swelling. When the invader has been defeated, there is no longer sufficient antigen to maintain B and T cells in an activated state. At this point, most B and T cells die from exhaustion or from lack of stimulation, and the swelling in your lymph nodes goes away.

You may also know that when surgeons remove a cancer from some organ in the body, they generally inspect the lymph nodes that drain the lymph from that organ. If they find cancer cells in the draining lymph nodes, it is an indication that the cancer has begun to metastasize via the lymphatic system to other parts of the body, the first stop being the nearby lymph nodes.

Peyer's patches

Back in the late seventeenth century, a Swiss anatomist, Johann Peyer, noticed patches of smooth cells embedded in the villi-covered cells that line the small intestine. We now know that these "Peyer's patches" are examples of mucosal-associated lymphoid tissues (MALT) which function as secondary lymphoid organs. Peyer's patches begin to develop before birth, and an adult human has about 200 of them. Here is a diagram that shows the basic features of a Peyer's patch.

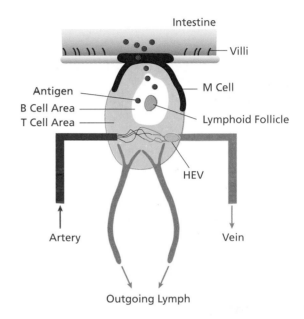

Peyer's patches have high endothelial venules through which lymphocytes can enter from the blood, and, of course, there are outgoing lymphatics that drain lymph away from these tissues. However, unlike lymph nodes, there are no incoming lymphatics that bring lymph into Peyer's patches. So if there are no incoming lymphatics, how does antigen enter this secondary lymphoid organ?

Do you see that smooth cell which crowns the Peyer's patch – the one that doesn't have "hairs" (villi) on it? That is called an "M" cell. These remarkable cells are not coated with mucus, so they are, by design, easily accessible to microorganisms that inhabit the intestine. They are "sampling" cells which specialize in transporting antigen from the interior (lumen) of the small intestine into the tissues beneath the M cell. To accomplish this feat, M cells enclose intestinal antigens in vesicles (endosomes). These endosomes are then transported <u>through</u> the M cell, and their contents are spit out into the tissues that surround the small intestine. So, **whereas lymph** nodes sample antigens from the lymph, Peyer's patches sample antigens from the intestine – and they do it by transporting these antigens through M cells.

Antigen that has been collected by M cells can be carried by the lymph to the lymph nodes that drain the Peyer's patches. Also, if the collected antigen is opsonized by complement or antibodies, it can be captured by follicular dendritic cells in lymphoid follicles that are below the M cells. In fact, except for its unusual method of acquiring antigen, a Peyer's patch is quite similar to a lymph node, with high endothelial venules to admit B and T cells, and special areas where these cells congregate.

Recently it was discovered that M cells are quite selective about the antigens they transport, so M cells don't just take "sips" of whatever is currently in the intestine (how disgusting!). Indeed, these cells only transport antigens that can bind to molecules on the surface of the M cell. This selectivity makes perfect sense. The whole idea of the M cell and the Peyer's patch is to help initiate an immune response to pathogens that invade via the intestinal tract. But for a pathogen to be troublesome, it has to be able to bind to cells that line the intestines and gain entry into the tissues below. So the minimum requirement for a microbe to be dangerous is that it be able to bind to the surface of an intestinal cell. In contrast, most of the stuff we eat will just pass through the intestine in various stages of digestion without binding to anything. Consequently, by ignoring all the "non-binders," M cells concentrate the efforts of a Peyer's patch on potential pathogens, and help avoid activating the immune system in response to innocuous food antigens.

The spleen

The final secondary lymphoid organ on our tour is the spleen. This organ is located between an artery and a vein, and it functions as a blood filter. Each time your heart pumps, about 5% of its output goes through your spleen. Consequently, it only takes about half an hour for your spleen to screen all the blood in your body for pathogens.

As with Peyer's patches, there are no lymphatics that bring lymph into the spleen. However, in contrast to lymph nodes and Peyer's patches, where entry of B and T cells from the blood occurs only via high endothelial venules, the spleen is like an "open-house party" in which everything in the blood is invited to enter. Here is a schematic diagram of one of the filter units that make up the spleen.

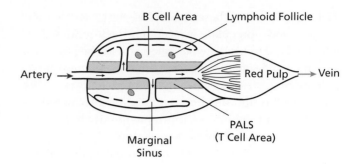

When blood enters from the splenic artery, it is diverted out to the marginal sinuses from which it percolates through the body of the spleen before it is collected into the splenic vein. The marginal sinuses are lined with macrophages that clean up the blood by phagocytosing cell debris and foreign invaders. As they ride along with the blood, naive B cells and T cells are temporarily retained in different areas – T cells in a region called the periarteriolar lymphocyte sheath (PALS) that surrounds the central arteriole, and B cells in the region between the PALS and the marginal sinuses.

Of course, since the spleen has no lymphatics to transport dendritic cells from the tissues, you might ask, "Where do the antigen presenting cells in the spleen come from?" The answer is that the marginal sinuses, where the blood first enters the spleen, is home to "resident" dendritic cells. These cells take up antigens from invaders in the blood and use them to prepare a class II MHC display. Resident dendritic cells also can be infected by pathogens in the blood, and can use their class I MHC molecules to display these antigens. Once activated, these dendritic cells travel to the PALS where T cells have gathered. So although the dendritic cells which present antigens to T cells in the spleen are travelers, their journey is relatively short compared with that of their cousins which travel to lymph nodes from a battle being waged in the tissues.

Helper T cells that have been activated by APCs in the PALS then move into the lymphoid follicles of the spleen to give help to B cells. You know the rest.

THE LOGIC OF SECONDARY LYMPHOID ORGANS

By now, I'm sure you have caught on to what Mother Nature is doing here. **Each secondary lymphoid organ is strategically positioned to intercept invaders that enter** the body by different routes. If the skin is punctured and the tissues become infected, an immune response is generated in the lymph nodes that drain those tissues. If you eat contaminated food, an immune response is initiated in the Peyer's patches that line your small intestine. If you are invaded by blood-borne pathogens, your spleen is there to filter them out and to fire up the immune response. And if an invader enters via your respiratory tract, another set of secondary lymphoid organs that includes your tonsils is there to defend you.

Not only are the secondary lymphoid organs strategically positioned, they provide a setting that is conducive to the mobilization of weapons that are appropriate to the kinds of invaders they are most likely to encounter. Exactly how this works isn't clear yet. However, it is believed that the different cytokine environments of the various secondary lymphoid organs determine the local character of the immune response. For example, Peyer's patches specialize in turning out Th cells that secrete a Th2 profile of cytokines as well as B cells that secrete IgA antibodies – weapons that are perfect to defend against intestinal invaders. In contrast, if you are invaded by bacteria from a splinter in your toe, the lymph node behind your knee will produce Th1 cells and B cells that secrete IgG antibodies – weapons ideal for defending against bacteria.

Earlier, I characterized secondary lymphoid organs as dating bars where T cells, B cells, and APCs mingle in an attempt to find their partners. But in fact, it's even better than that. Secondary lymphoid organs actually function more like "dating services." Here's what I mean.

When men and women use a dating service to find a mate, they begin by filling out a questionnaire that gives information on their backgrounds and their goals. Then, a computer goes through all these questionnaires and tries to match up men and women who might be compatible. In this way, the odds of a man finding a woman who is "right" for him is greatly increased – because they have been preselected. This type of preselection also takes place in the secondary lymphoid organs. Here's how it works.

During our tour, we noted that the secondary lymphoid organs are "segregated," with separate areas for naive T cells and B cells. As the billions of Th cells pass through the T cell areas of secondary lymphoid organs, only a tiny fraction of these cells will be activated – those whose cognate antigens are displayed by the antigen presenting cells that also populate the T cell areas. The Th cells that do not find their antigens leave the secondary

lymphoid organs and continue to circulate. Only those lucky Th cells which are activated in the T cell area will proliferate and then travel to a developing germinal center to provide help to B cells. This makes perfect sense: allowing useless, non-activated Th cells to enter B cell areas would just clutter things up, and would decrease the chances that Th and B cells which are "right" for each other might get together.

Likewise, many B cells enter the B cell areas of secondary lymphoid organs, looking for their cognate antigen displayed by follicular dendritic cells. Most just pass on through without finding the antigen their receptors recognize. Those rare B cells which do find their "mates" are retained in the secondary lymphoid organs, and are allowed to interact with activated Th cells. So by preselecting lymphocytes in their respective areas of secondary lymphoid organs, Mother Nature insures that when Th cells and B cells eventually do meet, they will have the maximum chance of finding their "mates" – just like a dating service.

Although preselecting Th and B cells before they get together is a good idea, the compartmentalization of lymphocytes in the secondary lymphoid organs does raise one problem. Activation of a naive B cell by an activated Th cell involves cell–cell contact during which the CD40L protein on the Th cell binds to the CD40 protein on the B cell. However, while this interaction between CD40L and CD40 is taking place, the engaged CD40L protein is rapidly taken into the interior of the Th cell and degraded. Pretty soon, the Th cell doesn't have enough CD40L left on its surface to provide help to B cells. In effect, the Th cell "runs out of gas." To "refill its tank," a Th cell must be restimulated. If this occurs, more CD40L proteins will be produced and transported to the surface of the Th cell, and the cell will be back in business. The problem, however, is that when the Th cell runs out of gas, it is no longer in the T cell zone, where the APCs that originally provided stimulation reside. So how does the Th cell get restimulated?

When B cells bind their cognate antigen displayed on follicular dendritic cells, the protein is taken into the B cell, cut into fragments, and presented by class II MHC molecules on the B cell surface. And once a B cell has been activated, it also expresses B7 proteins on its surface. Consequently, an activated B cell has all the goodies required to function as an APC and to restimulate helper T cells that have run out of gas. So, in a lymphoid follicle, Th cells and B cells do a "dance" in which the Th cell provides the co-stimulation (CD40L) required to

activate the B cell, and the B cell provides the presented antigen and co-stimulation (B7) required to "recharge" the T cell.

It is important to note that during this dance, the part of the protein which the B cell recognizes (the B cell epitope) usually is different from the part of the protein that the Th cells recognizes (the T cell epitope). A B cell's receptors bind to a portion of a protein which has the right shape to "fit" its receptors. The entire protein is then taken into the cell and cut up. Only those fragments of the protein which fit into the groove of a class II MHC molecule will be displayed on the B cell surface to activate the helper T cell. These fragments may be, but generally are not, cut from the same part of the protein that the B cell's receptors recognize. Said another way, the B cell epitope and the T cell epitope are "linked" – because they are from the same protein. But these epitopes usually are different.

LYMPHOCYTE TRAFFICKING

So far, we've talked about the secondary lymphoid organs in which B and T cells meet to do their activation thing, but I haven't said much about how these cells know to go there. Immunologists call this process "lymphocyte trafficking." In a human, about 500 billion lymphocytes circulate each day through the various secondary lymphoid organs. However, these cells don't just wander around. They follow a carefully orchestrated traffic pattern which maximizes their chances of encountering an invader. Importantly, **the traffic patterns of virgin and experienced lymphocytes are different**. Let's look first at the travels of a virgin T cell.

T cells begin life in the bone marrow and are educated in the thymus (lots more on this subject in Lecture 9). When they emerge from the thymus, virgin T cells express a mixture of cellular adhesion molecules on their surface. These function as "passports" for travel to any of the secondary lymphoid organs. For example, virgin T cells have a molecule called L-selectin on their surface that can bind to its adhesion partner, GlyCAM-1, which is found on the high endothelial venules of lymph nodes. This is their "lymph node passport." Virgin T cells also express an integrin molecule, $\alpha4\beta7$, whose adhesion partner, MadCAM-1, is found on the high endothelial venules of Peyer's patches and the lymph nodes that drain the tissues around the intestines (the mesenteric lymph nodes). So this integrin is their passport to the gut

region. Equipped with an array of adhesion molecules, inexperienced T cells circulate through all of the secondary lymphoid organs. This makes sense: the genes for a T cell's receptors are assembled by randomly selecting gene segments – so there is no telling where in the body a given naive T cell will encounter its cognate antigen.

In the secondary lymphoid organs, virgin T cells pass through fields of antigen presenting cells in the T cell areas. If they do not see their cognate antigens advertised there, they re-enter the blood either via the lymph or directly (in the case of the spleen), and continue to recirculate, making a complete circuit every 12 to 24 hours. A naive T cell can continue doing this circulation thing for quite some time, but after about six weeks, if the T cell has not encountered its cognate antigen presented by an MHC molecule, it will die by apoptosis, lonely and unsatisfied. In contrast, those lucky T cells that do find their antigen are activated in the secondary lymphoid organs. These are now "experienced" T cells.

Experienced T cells also carry passports, but they are "restricted passports," because, during activation, expression of certain adhesion molecules on the T cell surface is increased, whereas expression of others is decreased. This modulation of cellular adhesion molecule expression is not random. There's a plan here. In fact, **the cellular adhesion molecules that activated T cells express depend on where these T cells were activated.** For example, T cells activated in a Peyer's patch will express high levels of $\alpha4\beta7$ (the gut-specific integrin), and low levels of L-selectin (the more general, high endothelial venule adhesion molecule). As a result, T cells activated in Peyer's patches tend to return to Peyer's patches. Thus, **when activated T cells recirculate, they usually exit the blood and re-enter the same type of secondary lymphoid organ in which they originally encountered antigen.** This restricted traffic pattern is quite logical. After all, there is no use having experienced helper T cells recirculate to the lymph node behind your knee if your intestines have been invaded. Certainly not. You want those experienced helper T cells to get right back to the tissues that underlie your intestines to be restimulated and to provide help. So **by equipping activated T cells with restricted passports, Mother Nature insures that these cells will go back to where they are most likely to re-encounter their cognate antigens – be it in a Peyer's patch, a lymph node, or a tonsil.**

Now, of course, you don't want T cells to just go round and round. You also want them to exit the blood at sites of infection so that CTLs can kill pathogen-infected cells and Th cells can provide cytokines that amplify the immune response and recruit even more warriors from the blood. To make this happen, **experienced T cells also carry "combat passports" (adhesion molecules) which direct them to exit the blood at places where invaders have started an infection. These T cells employ the same "roll, sniff, stop, exit" technique that neutrophils use to leave the blood and enter inflamed tissues.** For example, T cells that gained their experience in the mucosa express an integrin molecule, $\alpha E\beta 7$, which has as its adhesion partner an addressin molecule that is expressed on inflamed mucosal blood vessels. As a result, T cells that have the right "training" to deal with mucosal invaders will seek out mucosal tissues which have been infected. In these tissues, chemokines given off by the soldiers at the front help direct T cells to the battle by binding to the chemokine receptors that appeared on the surface of the T cells during activation.

In summary, **naive T cells have passports that allow them to visit all the secondary lymphoid organs, but not sites of inflammation. This traffic pattern brings the entire collection of virgin T cells into contact (in the secondary lymphoid organs) with invaders that may have entered the body at any point, and greatly increases the probability that virgin T cells will be activated.** The reason that virgin T cells don't carry passports to battle sites is that they couldn't do anything there anyway – they must be activated first.

In contrast to virgin T cells, experienced T cells have restricted passports that encourage them to return to the same type of secondary lymphoid organ as the one in which they gained their experience. By recirculating preferentially to the kind of organ in which they first encountered antigen, T cells are more likely to be restimulated or to find CTLs and B cells that have encountered the same invader and need their help.

Activated T cells also have passports that allow them to exit the blood at sites of infection, enabling CTLs to kill infected cells and Th cells to provide appropriate cytokines to direct the battle. This marvelous "postal system," made up of cellular adhesion molecules and chemokines, insures delivery of the right weapons to the sites where they are needed.

B cell trafficking is roughly similar to T cell trafficking. **Like virgin T cells, virgin B cells also have passports that admit them to the complete range of secondary lymphoid organs. However, experienced B cells don't tend to be as migratory as experienced T cells. Most just settle down in secondary lymphoid organs or in the bone marrow, produce antibodies, and let these antibodies do the traveling.**

WHY MOTHERS KISS THEIR BABIES

Have you ever wondered why mothers kiss their babies? It's something they all do, you know. Most of the barnyard animals also kiss their babies, although in that case we call it licking. I'm going to tell you why they do it.

The immune system of a newborn human is not very well developed. In fact, production of IgG antibodies doesn't begin until a few months after birth. Fortunately, IgG antibodies from the mother's blood can cross the placenta into the fetus's blood, so a newborn has this "passive immunity" from mother to help tide him over. The newborn can also receive another type of passive immunity: IgA antibodies from mother's milk. During lactation, plasma B cells migrate to a mother's breasts and produce IgA antibodies that are secreted into the milk. This works great, because most pathogens that a baby encounters enter through his mouth or nose, travel to his intestines, and cause diarrhea. By drinking mother's milk that is rich in IgA antibodies, the baby's digestive tract is coated with antibodies that can intercept these pathogens.

When you think about it, however, a mother has been exposed to many different pathogens during her life, and the antibodies she makes to most of these will not be of any use to the infant. For example, it is likely that the mother has antibodies that recognize the Epstein–Barr virus that causes mononucleosis, but her child probably won't be exposed to this virus until he is a teenager. So wouldn't it be great if a mother could somehow provide antibodies that recognize the particular pathogens that her baby is encountering – and not provide antibodies that the baby has no use for? Well, that's exactly what happens.

When a mother kisses her baby, she "samples" those pathogens that are on the baby's face – the ones the baby is about to ingest. These samples are taken up by the mother's secondary lymphoid organs (e.g., her tonsils), and memory B cells specific for those pathogens are reactivated. These B cells then traffic to the mother's breasts where they produce a ton of antibodies – the very antibodies the baby needs for protection!

THOUGHT QUESTIONS

1. What are the functions of the various secondary lymphoid organs?

2. Make a table for each of the secondary lymphoid organs we discussed (lymph node, Peyer's patch, and spleen) which lists how antigen, B cells, and T cells enter and leave these organs.

3. In the T cell areas of secondary lymphoid organs, activated dendritic cells and Th cells interact. What goes on during this "dance"?

4. In the lymphoid follicles of secondary lymphoid organs, B cells and Th cells interact. What goes on during this "dance"?

5. What is the advantage of having virgin T cells circulate through all the secondary lymphoid organs?

6. What is the advantage of having experienced T cells circulate through selected secondary lymphoid organs?

Restraining the Immune System

REVIEW

In the last lecture, we visited three secondary lymphoid organs: a lymph node, a Peyer's patch, and the spleen. Secondary lymphoid organs are strategically situated to intercept invaders that breach the physical barriers and enter the tissues and the blood. Because of their locations, they play critical roles in immunity by creating an environment in which antigen, antigen presenting cells, and lymphocytes can gather to initiate an immune response.

B and T cells gain access to a lymph node either from the blood (by passing between specialized high endothelial cells) or via the lymph. Antigen can enter a lymph node with lymph drained from the tissues, so this organ functions as a lymph filter that intercepts invaders. In addition, antigen can be carried to a lymph node as cargo aboard an antigen presenting cell. In contrast, antigen is transported into a Peyer's patch through specialized M cells that sample antigen from the intestine. This antigen can interact with B and T cells that have entered the Peyer's patch via high endothelial venules, or it can travel with the lymph to the lymph nodes that drain the Peyer's patch. Thus, a Peyer's patch is a secondary lymphoid organ designed to deal with pathogens attempting to breach the intestinal mucosal barrier. Finally, we talked about the spleen, a secondary lymphoid organ that is quite different from either a lymph node or a Peyer's patch in that it has no incoming lymphatics and no high endothelial venules. As a result of this "plumbing," antigen and lymphocytes must enter the spleen via the blood. This construction makes the spleen an ideal blood filter that intercepts blood-borne pathogens.

Virgin helper T cells travel though the blood, and enter the secondary lymphoid organs. If a Th cell does not encounter its cognate antigen displayed by an APC in the T cell zone, it exits the organ via the lymph or blood (depending on the organ), and visits other secondary lymphoid organs in search of its cognate antigen. On the other hand, if during its visit to a secondary lymphoid organ, a Th cell does find its cognate antigen displayed by class II MHC molecules on a dendritic cell, it becomes activated and proliferates. Most of the progeny then exit the secondary lymphoid organ and travel again through the lymph and the blood. These "experienced" Th cells have adhesion molecules on their surface that encourage them to re-enter the same type of secondary lymphoid organ in which they were activated (e.g., a Peyer's patch or a peripheral lymph node). This restricted recirculation following initial activation and proliferation spreads activated Th cells around to those secondary lymphoid organs in which B cells or CTLs are likely to be waiting for their help. Recirculating Th cells also can exit the blood vessels that run through sites of inflammation. There Th cells provide cytokines which strengthen the reaction of the innate and adaptive systems to the attack, and which help recruit even more immune system cells from the blood.

Virgin killer T cells also circulate through the blood, lymph, and secondary lymphoid organs. They can be activated if they encounter their cognate antigen displayed by class I MHC molecules on the surfaces of antigen presenting cells in the T cell zones of secondary lymphoid organs. Like experienced Th cells, experienced CTLs can proliferate and recirculate to secondary lymphoid organs to be restimulated, or they can leave the circulation and enter inflamed tissues to kill cells infected with viruses or other parasites (e.g., intracellular bacteria).

Virgin B cells also travel to secondary lymphoid organs, looking for their cognate antigens. If they are unsuccessful,

REVIEW (continued)

they continue circulating through the blood, lymph, and secondary lymphoid organs until they either find their mates or die of neglect. In the lymphoid follicles of the secondary lymphoid organs, a lucky B cell that finds the antigen to which its receptors can bind will migrate to the border of the lymphoid follicle. There, if it receives the required co-stimulation from an activated helper T cell, the B cell will be activated, and will proliferate to produce many more B cells that can recognize the same antigen. All this activity converts a primary lymphoid follicle, which is just a loose collection of follicular dendritic cells and B cells, into a "germinal center" in which B cells proliferate and mature. In a germinal center, B cells may "class switch" to produce IgA, IgG, or IgE antibodies, and they may undergo somatic hypermutation to increase the average affinity of their receptors for antigen. Most of these B cells become plasma cells and travel to the spleen or bone marrow, where they produce antibodies. Others recirculate to secondary lymphoid organs that are similar to the one in which they were activated. There they amplify the response by being restimulated to proliferate some more. Still other B cells go back to the resting state in the spleen or bone marrow to function as memory cells.

In summary, virgin B and T cells are equipped with adhesion molecules and chemokine receptors that promote travel to all secondary lymphoid organs, but which do not allow travel to inflamed tissues. As a result, the entire repertoire of BCRs and TCRs is brought together in the secondary lymphoid organs – where the probability is highest that they will encounter their cognate antigens in an environment appropriate for activation. Once activated, B and T cells express adhesion molecules that encourage them to travel back to the same type of secondary lymphoid organ in which they were originally activated. Experienced T cells also are awarded passports which allow them to exit the blood at sites of infection so that they can participate in the struggle against invaders.

The immune system evolved to provide a rapid and overwhelming response to invading pathogens. After all, most attacks by viruses or bacteria result in acute infections that either are quickly dealt with by the immune system (in a matter of days or weeks) or which overwhelm the immune system and kill you. Built into this system are positive feedback loops in which various immune system players work together to get each other fired up. However, once an invasion has been repulsed, these feedback loops must be broken, and the system must be turned off. In addition, there are times when a vigorous response to an invasion simply is not appropriate, and in these situations, the immune system must be restrained in order to prevent irreparable damage to our bodies.

Until recently, immunologists spent most of their effort trying to understand how the immune system gets turned on, and great progress has been made in that area. Now, however, many immunologists have begun to focus on the equally important question of how the system is "restrained," so that it doesn't exert excessive force or continue to mobilize and deploy weapons even after an invader has been vanquished.

AVOIDING OVERREACTION

Our intestines are home to about 100 trillion bacteria of at least 1000 different types. Most of these bacteria are "commensal" (from the Greek, meaning roughly to "eat at the same table"). Indeed, they are indispensable for our digestion because they function to partially degrade the polysaccharides in the food we eat. Some of these commensal bacteria also produce vitamins which we require for survival. Moreover, because these "friendly" bacteria are so well adapted to live in our intestines, they can help protect us from dangerous bacteria by out-competing the bad guys for available resources and physical niches. So hosting these commensal bacteria can be beneficial. However, the single layer of epithelial cells which separates them from the tissues that surround the intestines is so thin, its area is so vast (about 200 square meters), and the bacteria are so numerous that, even under normal conditions, some of them will breach this barrier and enter the tissues.

This situation poses a real dilemma for the immune system. If it reacts too strongly to these friendly bacteria, the tissues surrounding your intestines would be in a constant state of inflammation – which would cause diarrhea and all sorts of other problems. On the other hand, if these errant commensal bacteria are not dealt with, they could enter the blood stream and cause a life-threatening, systemic infection. Moreover, pathogenic bacteria, which are not so friendly, can also breach the intestinal barrier, and the immune system must react decisively against these dangerous invaders. What this means is that the immune system must somehow know how to deal gently with intestinal bacteria that are not inherently dangerous, but harshly with those which can do serious harm. How the immune system avoids "over-exuberance" is currently the subject of intense investigation, and some clues about how the immune system exercises appropriate restraint have emerged.

Experiments with mice indicate that special macrophages patrol the tissues which underlie the intestinal wall. Although these warriors phagocytose invading bacteria, they usually do not give off cytokines which would signal a full-blown attack. IgA is the major antibody class produced by B cells in these tissues, and these antibodies can efficiently bind to invading bacteria and usher them back out of the tissues into the intestine. However, the Fc portion of an IgA antibody cannot bind with high affinity to receptors on immune system cells to trigger an inflammatory response – as, for example, IgG antibodies would do. So, **under normal conditions, macrophages and IgA antibodies act with restraint to deal with commensal bacteria which occasionally enter the tissues from the intestines.**

ATTENUATING THE IMMUNE RESPONSE

We generally think of Th cells as providing help to turn the immune system on, but recently, **another type of CD4+ T cell has been discovered which actually helps turn the system off: the inducible regulatory T cell (iTreg).** These cells are called "regulatory" because, instead of producing cytokines such as TNF and IFN-γ which activate the immune system, they produce cytokines such as IL-10 and TGFβ that help restrain the system. When TGFβ binds to receptors on T cells, it reduces the proliferation rate of these cells and makes killer T cells less vicious killers. IL-10 works by binding to its receptors on T cells and blocking co-stimulatory signals (e.g., signals transmitted through CD28). This makes it more difficult to activate these cells, and decreases their rate of proliferation. These regulatory T cells are termed "inducible" because, **just as naive helper T cells can be encouraged to become Th1, Th2, or Th17 cells, naive Th cells can also be "induced" to become iTregs.** Here's the way this is thought to work.

Under non-battle conditions, when the integrity of the intestinal barrier has not been compromised, the epithelial cells that line the intestine produce the cytokine TGFβ. And when naive Th cells are activated in the Peyer's patches that underlie the intestine, they are encouraged by this cytokine to become iTregs. These T cells then give off cytokines which help keep the mucosal immune system "calmed down."

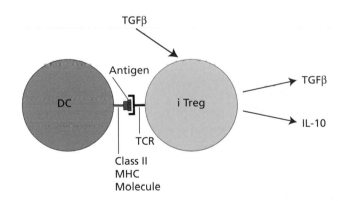

Now, you may remember that TGFβ is one of the cytokines that causes naive Th cells to become Th17 cells – cells which are skilled at orchestrating an inflammatory response to a bacterial or fungal invasion. So how does the immune system decide whether Th cells that are guarding against intestinal invaders should become iTregs and restrain the immune response, or become Th17 cells and "let the dogs out"? The answer to this question is not known for certain, but it appears, as you'd expect, that it is the dendritic cell which makes this decision. **If there is an invasion of pathogenic bacteria, dendritic cells begin to produce IL-6, which influences helper T cells to commit to becoming Th17 cells. If there is no**

real danger, and things just need to be kept calm, dendritic cells don't produce IL-6 – and naive Th cells, under the influence of tissue-produced TGFβ become iTregs. And how do dendritic cells know the difference between pathogenic and commensal bacteria? Nobody knows for sure, but it may have to do with receptors on dendritic cells which recognize pathogenic vs. commensal bacteria.

DEACTIVATING THE SYSTEM

The innate immune response is initiated when the receptors of cells such as macrophages detect either the molecular signatures of an invader or the results of an attack (e.g., dying cells). Likewise, the adaptive system is activated when T cells recognize antigens derived from invading pathogens that have been transported by dendritic cells to the secondary lymphoid organs. However, as the immune system gains the upper hand and invaders are destroyed, there will be less and less "invading antigen" present. Consequently, fewer innate system cells will be activated, and fewer dendritic cells will mature and travel with their cargo of battle antigens to secondary lymphoid organs. So as foreign antigen is eliminated, the level of activation of both the innate and adaptive systems decreases. This is the first step in deactivating the immune system.

Although the removal of foreign antigen is the most important factor in turning off the system, other mechanisms also help decrease the level of activation as the battle winds down. In Lecture 5, we discussed the B7 proteins which are expressed on the surface of antigen presenting cells, and which provide co-stimulation to T cells by plugging into receptors called CD28 on a T cell's surface. This interaction sets off a cascade of events within a T cell that reduces the total number of T cell receptors which must be crosslinked in order to activate the T cell, making activation more efficient. However, in addition to engaging stimulatory CD28 molecules, B7 proteins also can plug into another receptor on T cells called CTLA-4. In contrast to ligation of CD28, which increases activation, engagement of CTLA-4 represses activation by antagonizing the CD28 activation signal within the T cell. Moreover, because B7 binds to CTLA-4 with an affinity which is thousands of times higher than its affinity for CD28, CTLA-4 also suppresses activation by occupying B7 molecules so they cannot bind to CD28.

Most human T cells display CD28 on their surface, so it is always available to assist with activation. In contrast, most of a naive T cell's CTLA-4 is stored inside the cell. Once these T cells have been activated, however, more and more CTLA-4 is moved from these intracellular reservoirs to the cell surface where, because of its higher affinity, CTLA-4 eventually out-competes CD28 for B7 binding. As a result, **early in an infection, B7 binds to CD28 and acts as a co-stimulator. Then, after the battle has been raging for a while, B7 binds mainly to CTLA-4, making it harder, instead of easier, for these T cells to be reactivated, and helping to shut down the adaptive immune response.**

LIFE IS SHORT

As a consequence of the removal of foreign antigen and the subsequent cessation of activation, the immune system will stop making weapons which can defend against a banished invader. Although this is an important step in turning off the immune response after an attack has ended, many of the weapons made during the struggle will remain at the battle site, and these stockpiles of obsolete weapons must somehow be "decommissioned."

Fortunately, many of the weapons of the immune system only live for a short time. For example, during a major invasion, huge numbers of neutrophils are recruited from the blood, but these cells are programed to die after a few days. Likewise, natural killer cells have a half-life of only about a week. Consequently, once recruitment ceases, the stockpiles of neutrophils and NK cells are quickly depleted. Moreover, because natural killer cells supply IFN-γ to help keep macrophages fired up, when NK cells die off, macrophages tend to go back to a resting state.

Dendritic cells, once they reach a lymph node, only live about a week, and plasma B cells die after about five days of hard labor. Consequently, as the activation of Th and B cells wanes, the number of plasma B cells specific for an invader declines rapidly. Moreover, the antibodies which plasma cells produce have short lifetimes, with the longest lived (the IgG class) having a half-life of only about three weeks. As a result, once plasma B cells stop being produced, the number of invader-specific antibodies drops rapidly.

EXHAUSTION

So part of the problem of disposing of obsolete weapons is solved by making many of these weapons short-lived. T cells, however, are an important exception to this "rule." In contrast to cells like neutrophils, which are programmed to self-destruct after a short time on the job, T cells are designed to live a long time. The reason for this is that naive T cells must circulate again and again through the secondary lymphoid organs, looking for their particular antigen on display – so it would be extremely wasteful if T cells were short-lived. On the other hand, once T cells have been activated, have proliferated in response to an attack, and have defeated the invader, the longevity of T cells could be a major problem. Indeed, at the height of some viral attacks, more than 10% of all our T cells recognize that particular virus. If most of these cells were not eliminated, our bodies would soon fill up with obsolete

T cells that could only defend us against invaders from the past. Fortunately, Mother Nature recognized this problem and invented "activation-induced cell death" (AICD) – a way of eliminating obsolete T cells after they have been restimulated many times in the course of a battle. Here's how this works.

CTLs have proteins called Fas ligand that are prominently displayed on their surface, and one way they kill is by plugging this protein into its binding partner, Fas, which is present on the surface of target cells. When these proteins connect, the target is triggered to commit suicide by apoptosis. Virgin T cells are "wired" so that they are insensitive to ligation of their Fas proteins. However, when T cells are activated and then reactivated many times during an attack, their internal wiring changes. When this happens, they become increasingly more sensitive to ligation of their Fas proteins either by their own Fas ligand proteins or by Fas ligand proteins on other T cells. This feature makes these "exhausted" T cells targets for Fas-mediated killing – either through suicide or homicide. In fact, once an invader has been vanquished, more than 90% of the T cells which responded to the attack usually die off. By this mechanism, activation-induced cell death (AICD) eliminates T cells which have been repeatedly activated, and makes room for new T cells that can protect us from the next microbes which might try to do us in.

In summary, the dependence of continued activation on the presence of foreign antigen, the effect of negative regulators of activation such as CTLA-4, the short lifetimes of many immune warriors, and activation-induced death of "fatigued" T cells all work together to help turn the immune system off and to dispose of obsolete weapons once a battle has been won. These mechanisms combine to "reset" the system after each infection, so that it will be ready to deal with the next attack.

THOUGHT QUESTIONS

1. What special features of the immune system in the tissues which surround the intestines help avoid an overreaction to commensal bacteria?

2. Why are IgA antibodies called "passive" antibodies?

3. Why are inducible T regulatory cells (iTregs) important, and how do they function?

4. Why doesn't the interaction between B7 proteins on APCs and CTLA-4 proteins prevent the activation of naive T cells?

5. Wouldn't it be better just to activate fewer T cells, so that "excess" T cells would not have to be destroyed by activation-induced cell death? Why not?

LECTURE 9

Tolerance Induction and MHC Restriction

REVIEW

Although the immune defense usually reacts quickly and decisively against dangerous invaders, there are also situations when the system must act with restraint. For example, commensal bacteria which breach the intestinal barrier must be dealt with gently because they do not pose a great threat. Consequently, macrophages which guard the tissues that surround the intestines are "programed" to phagocytose commensal bacteria without giving off cytokines that would signal a dangerous attack. Likewise, the predominate antibodies which defend these areas are of the IgA class. These antibodies act "passively" by binding invaders and ushering them back out into the intestines – without causing inflammation. In addition, inducible regulatory T cells (iTregs) reside in the tissues beneath the intestines. These helper T cells secrete cytokines designed to keep the intestinal immune system "calm" when we are not threatened by dangerous invaders.

Once an invasion has been repulsed, the immune response must be "turned off," and most of the weapons intended for use against that particular invader must be "decommissioned." Otherwise, the immune system would quickly fill up with weapons which only could protect against past invaders or which were stockpiled at the wrong locations to defend against future attacks. The first step in turning off the system is to reduce the level of activation, so that the production of new weapons slows down and finally ceases. The activation level is mainly controlled by the amount of foreign antigen present. Consequently, as invaders are destroyed, less foreign antigen remains, the activation level drops, and fewer new weapons are produced and deployed. In addition, when T cells have been activated, they begin to express the CTLA-4 protein on their surface. In contrast to CD28, which makes activation of T cells easier when it is ligated by B7 proteins expressed by antigen presenting cells, CTLA-4 is a negative regulator of activation. Indeed, ligation of CTLA-4 proteins on activated T cells negates the positive effects of CD28 ligation. This makes it harder for these T cells to be reactivated, and helps decrease the overall level of T cell activation.

Although curtailing the production of new weapons is the first step in turning off the immune response, something also must be done to eliminate most of the weapons which already have been manufactured and deployed. Fortunately, many of the weapons of the innate and adaptive systems have short lifetimes. Consequently, once production ceases, most of the weapons that were produced earlier in the infection are eliminated. In addition, T cells that have been repeatedly activated during the battle become increasingly susceptible to killing by ligation of their Fas proteins. As a result, these exhausted cells succumb to activation-induced cell death.

The subject of this lecture is one of the most exciting in all of immunology. Part of that excitement arises because, although a huge amount of research has been done on tolerance of self and MHC restriction, there are still many unanswered questions. What really makes this topic so interesting, however, is that it is so important. B cells and T cells must "learn" not to recognize our own "self" antigens as dangerous, for otherwise we would all die of autoimmune disease. In addition, T cells must be "restricted" to recognize self MHC, so that the attention of T cells will be focused on MHC-peptide complexes – and not on unpresented antigen.

THE THYMUS

T cells first learn tolerance of self in the thymus, a small organ located just below the neck. This process usually is called "central tolerance induction." Like the spleen, the thymus has no incoming lymphatics, so cells enter the thymus from the blood. However, in contrast to the spleen, which welcomes anything that is in the blood, entry of cells into the thymus is quite restricted. It is believed that immature T cells from the bone marrow enter the thymus from the blood, somewhere in the middle of the thymus. However, exactly how this happens is not understood, because the high endothelial cells that allow lymphocytes to exit the blood into secondary lymphoid organs are missing from the thymus. Antigens also are thought to enter from the blood, but again, the rules that govern their entry are unclear.

What <u>is</u> known is that the T cells enter the thymus from the bone marrow "in the nude": they don't express CD4, CD8, or a TCR. After entry, these cells migrate to the outer region of the thymus (the cortex) and begin to proliferate.

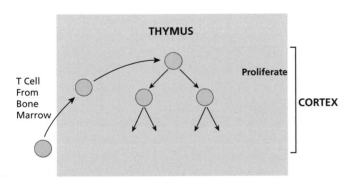

About this time, some of the cells start to rearrange the gene segments that encode the α and β chains of the TCR. If these rearrangements are successful, a T cell begins to express low levels of the TCR and its associated, accessory proteins (the CD3 protein complex). As a result, these formerly nude cells soon are "dressed" with CD4, CD8, and TCR molecules on their surface. Because these T cells express both CD4 and CD8 co-receptor molecules, they are called double positive (DP) cells.

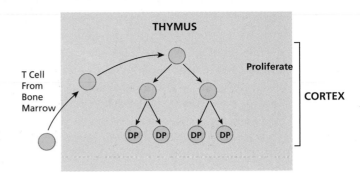

During this "reverse striptease," another important change takes place. When the T cell was naked, it was resistant to death by apoptosis, because it expressed little or no Fas antigen (which can trigger death when ligated), and because it expressed high levels of Bcl-2 (a cellular protein that protects against apoptosis). In contrast, **a "fully dressed" T cell of the thymic cortex expresses high levels of Fas on its surface and produces very little Bcl-2. Consequently, it is exquisitely sensitive to signals that can trigger death by apoptosis. It is in this highly vulnerable condition that a T cell is tested for tolerance of self and MHC restriction. If it fails either test, it will die.**

MHC RESTRICTION

The process of testing T cells for MHC restriction is usually referred to as "positive selection." The "examiners" here are epithelial cells in the cortical region of the thymus, and the question a cortical epithelial cell asks of a T cell is: do you have receptors that recognize one of the self MHC molecules which I am expressing on my surface? The correct answer is, "Yes, I do!" for if its TCRs do not recognize any of these self MHC molecules, the T cell dies.

When I say "self" MHC, I simply mean those MHC molecules which are expressed by the person (or mouse) who "owns" this thymus. Yes, this does seem like a no-brainer – that my T cells would be tested in my thymus on my MHC molecules – but immunologists like to emphasize this point by saying "self MHC."

The MHC molecules on the surface of the cortical epithelial cells are actually loaded with peptides, so what a TCR really recognizes is the combination of a self MHC molecule and its associated peptide. These peptides represent a "sampling" of the proteins that are being made by the cortical epithelial cells (displayed by class I MHC molecules) plus a "sampling" of all the proteins which the cortical epithelial cells have picked up from the environment within the thymus (displayed by class II MHC molecules).

THE LOGIC OF MHC RESTRICTION

Let's pause for a moment between exams to ask an important question: why do T cells need to be tested to be sure that they can recognize peptides presented by self MHC molecules? After all, most humans complete their lifetimes without ever seeing "foreign" MHC molecules (e.g., on a transplanted organ), so MHC restriction can't be about discriminating between your MHC molecules and mine. No, MHC restriction has nothing to do with foreign versus self – it's all about focus. As we discussed in Lecture 4, we want the system to be set up so that T cells focus on antigens that are presented by MHC molecules. However, T cell receptors are made by mixing and matching gene segments, so they are incredibly diverse. As a result, it is certain that in the collection of TCRs expressed on T cells, there will be many which recognize unpresented antigens, just as a B cell's receptors do. These T cells must be eliminated. Otherwise the wonderful system of antigen presentation by MHC molecules won't work. So the reason positive selection (MHC restriction) is so important is that it sets up a system in which all mature T cells will have TCRs that recognize antigen presented by MHC molecules.

TESTING FOR TOLERANCE OF SELF

During or slightly after positive selection takes place in the cortex of the thymus, T cells stop displaying either one or the other of the co-receptor molecules, CD4 or CD8. As you'd predict, these cells are then called single positive (SP) cells. How a T cell "chooses" to display CD4 co-receptors or CD8 co-receptors is still a mystery.

Those lucky T cells whose TCRs recognize self MHC plus peptide proceed from the thymic cortex to the central region of the thymus called the medulla. It is in the thymic medulla that the second test is administered: the test for tolerance of self. This exam is frequently referred to as "negative selection." Two types of cells pose this second question which "student" T cells must answer, and both cell types are different from the cortical thymic epithelial cells that tested T cells for MHC restriction.

The first type of cell that administers the exam for self tolerance is a thymic dendritic cell which has traveled to the thymus from the bone marrow. Although thymic DCs have the starfish-like shape that is characteristic of dendritic cells in general, they are different from either the antigen presenting dendritic cells or the follicular dendritic cells we have discussed previously.

The exam question posed by a thymic dendritic cell is: do you recognize any of the self peptides displayed by the MHC molecules on my surface? The correct answer is, "No way!" because T cells with receptors that do recognize the combination of MHC molecules and self peptides are deleted. The reason this second test, which eliminates T cells that could react against our own antigens, is so important is that if such self-reactive T cells were not deleted, autoimmune disease could result. For example, Th cells that recognize self antigens could help B cells make antibodies that would tag our own molecules (e.g., the insulin proteins in our blood) for destruction. In addition, CTLs could be produced that would attack our own cells.

One important feature of negative selection is that thymic dendritic cells only survive for a about a week in the thymus. Consequently, they only present what you might call "current" self antigen. This is really smart, because if foreign antigens were to reach the thymus (as they certainly can do during an infection), dendritic cells could use them for testing, just as if they were authentic self antigens. As a result, any maturing T cells that recognize the invader would be deleted for as long as thymic dendritic cells continued to present the foreign antigens. The short lifetime of thymic dendritic cells protects against this possibility, and allows T cells to be examined only on "new material." Once foreign antigens associated with an infection have been eliminated from the body, freshly made thymic dendritic cells will no longer present foreign antigen as self – and T cells that can recognize the invader will again survive negative selection.

One puzzle surrounding tolerance induction in the thymus has been that, in addition to the "shared" proteins which all cells produce, there are many proteins (estimates suggest several thousand) that are "tissue-specific." These are the proteins which give each organ or tissue type its identity. For example, there are proteins produced by the cells that make up your heart which are unique to this organ, and there are proteins made by kidney cells that are kidney-specific. So for tolerance testing in the thymus to be complete, tissue-specific proteins would need to be included in the "material" on which student T cells are tested. Otherwise, when killer T cells leave the thymus, some of them would surely encounter tissue-specific proteins to which they were not tolerant – and set about destroying your liver, your heart, or your kidneys. Not good.

When immunologists looked at the proteins made by thymic dendritic cells, they found that these cells do not express tissue-specific antigens – implying that T cells are not tested for tolerance to tissue-specific, self antigens. This potential defect in thymic tolerance induction was very disturbing, because it showed that there was something important about negative selection in the thymus which had not been fully understood.

Fortunately, this mystery has now been, at least partially, solved. **Immunologists have discovered a second type of cell that is involved in testing T cells for tolerance of self: medullary thymic epithelial cells.** These cells are cousins of the cortical thymic epithelial cells that test for MHC restriction, but they are different from those cells in a very interesting way: **medullary thymic epithelial cells express, in addition to the usual shared proteins, several thousand tissue-specific proteins.** It is now believed that medullary thymic epithelial cells are the source of the tissue-specific antigens which are used to test whether or not T cells are tolerant of these self antigens. I say "source," because it is not yet clear whether these cells actually do the testing, or whether they somehow transfer these antigens to thymic dendritic cells – which then do the testing. Also, it is not known whether medullary thymic epithelial cells express all of the tissue-specific proteins found in the body or just most of them. So there is still a lot of mystery surrounding the issue of tolerance to tissue-specific antigens.

Working together, thymic dendritic cells and medullary thymic epithelial cells might be able to present a relatively complete display of self antigens on class I MHC molecules in order to test killer T cells for self tolerance. After all, the job of class I MHC molecules is to display a sampling of all the proteins that a cell is making. In contrast, one might ask how the class II molecules on thymic dendritic cells could hope to display all of the possible self antigens in order to test Th cells for tolerance. This question arises because dendritic cells get the "raw material" they use for class II display by sampling proteins that are present in the environment outside the cell – and it is hard to imagine that the special environment within the thymus would contain all possible self antigens. Consequently, one would predict that many self antigens – those that were not "floating around" in the thymus – would be missed, and self reactive Th cells would result.

To solve this problem, what you'd like is a special examiner cell which could "break the law" and display, on class II MHC molecules, a sampling of all the proteins made by the cell (i.e., all the self antigens), just like class I MHC molecules do. Interestingly, the latest experiments suggest that medullary thymic epithelial cells are lawbreakers as far as class II display is concerned. Here's how this is thought to work.

Cells have evolved several mechanisms to help them deal with times of starvation when the raw materials required for the synthesis of cellular components are limiting. One such survival tool is a process called "autophagy." When cells are starving, they can enclose portions of their cytoplasm in a membrane, which then fuses with a lysosome. The cytoplasmic components (e.g., proteins) are then disassembled by lysosomal enzymes so that they can be reused. Immunologists have demonstrated that, at least in some medullary thymic epithelial cells, autophagy takes place all the time, and that a portion of the degraded proteins can be processed for display on class II MHC molecules. Thus, autophagy may provide the diverse source of self antigens required to eliminate most self-reactive helper T cells during negative selection.

GRADUATION

The final result of all this testing in the thymus is a T cell that has receptors which <u>do</u> recognize self MHC-peptide complexes presented by cortical thymic epithelial cells, but which do <u>not</u> recognize self antigens presented by MHC molecules on thymic dendritic cells or medullary thymic epithelial cells.

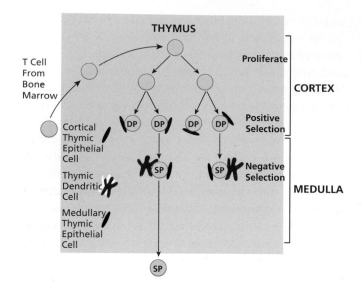

The "thymic graduates" that pass these tests express high levels (i.e., many molecules) of the T cell receptor on their surface, and either the CD4 or CD8 co-receptor, but not both. Each day in the thymus of a young person, about 60 million double positive cells are tested, but only about 2 million single positive cells exit the thymus. The rest die a horrible death by apoptosis, and are quickly eaten by macrophages in the thymus. Most students are not too thrilled about exams that last more than an hour, so I thought you might like to know that these tests take about two weeks! We're talking major exams here, where the life of each T cell hangs in the balance.

Interestingly, immunologists still don't know how these graduates leave the thymus. It may be via the lymph or the blood or by some combination of these two routes.

THE RIDDLE OF MHC RESTRICTION AND TOLERANCE INDUCTION

Now, if you've been paying close attention, you may be wondering how <u>any</u> T cells could possibly pass both exams. After all, to pass the test for MHC restriction, their TCRs must recognize MHC plus self peptide. Yet to pass the tolerance exam, their TCRs must <u>not</u> be able to recognize MHC plus self peptide. Doesn't it seem that the two exams would cancel each other out, allowing no T cells to pass? It certainly does, and this is the essence of the riddle of self tolerance: how can a T cell receptor possibly mediate both positive selection (MHC restriction) and negative selection (tolerance induction)? In fact, it is even more complicated than that, because once a T cell has

been educated in the thymus, its TCRs must be able to signal activation when they encounter invader-derived peptides presented by MHC molecules. So the question that vexes immunologists is: **how does the same TCR, when it engages MHC–peptide complexes, signal three, very different outcomes – positive selection, negative selection, or activation?**

Unfortunately, I can't answer this riddle (otherwise I'd be on my way to Sweden to pick up my Nobel Prize), but I can tell you the current thinking. Immunologists believe that the events leading to MHC restriction and tolerance induction are similar to those involved in the activation of T cells: cell-cell adhesion, TCR clustering, and co-stimulation. It is hypothesized that in the thymus, positive selection (survival) of T cells results from a <u>relatively weak</u> interaction between TCRs and MHC–self peptide displayed on cortical thymic epithelial cells. Negative selection (death) is induced by a <u>strong interaction</u> between TCRs and MHC–self peptide expressed on bone marrow-derived, thymic dendritic cells or medullary thymic epithelial cells. And activation of T cells after they leave the thymus results from a <u>strong interaction</u> between TCRs and MHC–peptide displayed by professional antigen presenting cells.

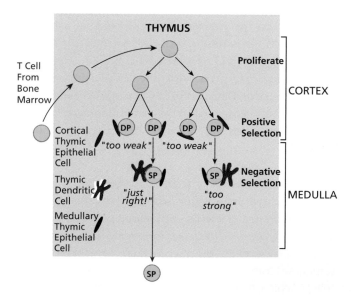

The question, of course, is what makes the effect of these three interactions of MHC–peptide with a T cell receptor so different – life, death, or activation? One key element appears to be the properties of the cell that "sends" the signal. In the case of MHC restriction, this is a cortical thymic epithelial cell. For tolerance induction, the cell is a bone marrow-derived dendritic cell or a medullary thymic epithelial cell. And for activation, the sender is a specialized antigen presenting cell. All these cells are very different, and it is likely that they differ in the cellular adhesion molecules they express, and in the number or type of MHC–peptide complexes they display on their surfaces. For example, it has been discovered that the proteasomes of cortical thymic epithelial cells are subtly different from the proteasomes of the cells that are responsible for negative selection. This could be expected to affect which self peptides are presented by these examiner cells. Such differences in adhesion molecules and MHC–peptide complexes could dramatically influence the strength of the signal that is sent through the T cell receptor. In addition, different types of cells are likely to express different mixtures of co-stimulatory molecules – and co-stimulatory signals could change the meaning of the signal that results from TCR–MHC–peptide engagements.

Not only are the cells that send the signals different, but the "receiver" (the T cell) also may change between exams. It is known that the number of TCRs on the surface of the T cell increases as the cell is educated, and it is also possible that the "wiring" within the T cell changes as the T cell matures. These differences in TCR density and signal processing could influence the interpretation of signals generated by the three types of sender cells.

Although many of the pieces of the MHC restriction/tolerance induction puzzle have been found, immunologists still have not been able to assemble them into a completely consistent picture. More work is required.

TOLERANCE BY IGNORANCE

Thankfully, most T cells with receptors which could recognize our own proteins are eliminated in the thymus. However, central tolerance is not foolproof. If it were, every single T cell would have to be tested on every possible self antigen in the thymus – and that's a lot to ask. The probability is great that T cells with receptors which have a <u>high affinity</u> for self antigens that are <u>abundant</u> in the thymus will be deleted there. However, T cells whose receptors have a low affinity for self antigens, or which recognize self antigens that are rare in the thymus, are less likely to be negatively selected. They may just "slip through the cracks" of central tolerance induction. Fortunately, the system has been set up to deal with this possibility.

Virgin T cells circulate through the secondary lymphoid organs, but are not allowed out into the tissues. This traffic pattern takes these virgins to the areas of the body where they are most likely to encounter APCs and be activated. However, the travel restriction that keeps virgin T cells out of the tissues also is important in maintaining self tolerance. The reason is that, as a rule, those self antigens which are abundant in the secondary lymphoid organs, where virgin lymphocytes are activated, also are abundant in the thymus, where T cells are tolerized. Therefore, as a result of the traffic pattern followed by virgin T cells, most T cells that could be activated by an abundant self antigen in the secondary lymphoid organs already will have been eliminated by seeing that same, abundant self antigen in the thymus.

Conversely, T cells whose receptors recognize self antigens that are relatively rare in the thymus may escape deletion there. However, these same antigens usually exist at such low concentrations in the secondary lymphoid organs that they do not activate potentially self-reactive T cells. Thus, although rare self antigens are present in the secondary lymphoid organs, and although T cells do have receptors which can recognize them, these T cells usually remain functionally "ignorant" of their presence – because the self antigens are too rare to trigger activation. Consequently, lymphocyte traffic patterns play a key role not only in insuring the efficient activation of the adaptive immune system, but also in preserving tolerance of self antigens.

TOLERANCE INDUCTION IN SECONDARY LYMPHOID ORGANS

Although the restricted traffic pattern of naive T cells usually protects them from exposure to self antigens which might activate them, this barrier to activation is not absolute. Occasionally, self antigens, which are too rare in the thymus to cause deletion of potentially autoreactive T cells, are released into the blood and lymphatic systems (e.g., as the result of an injury which causes tissue damage) in concentrations sufficient to activate previously ignorant T cells. But again, Mother Nature has figured out how to deal with this potential problem.

We have discussed how T cells that recognize self antigens in the thymus are eliminated to prevent autoimmunity, and until recently, it was believed that this was the only role of the thymus in tolerance induction. However, in the last few years, it has become clear that the thymus plays an additional important role in preventing autoimmunity. It is believed that a subset of thymic CD4+ T cells is selected (by an unknown mechanism) to become "natural" regulatory T cells (nTregs). This selection results in the expression of a gene called *Foxp3*, which is instrumental in conferring upon these nTreg cells their regulatory properties. After they are generated in the thymus, natural Tregs receive passports (adhesion molecules) which allow them to enter lymph nodes and other secondary lymphoid organs. Indeed, about 5% of all the CD4+ T cells in circulation are regulatory T cells. In the secondary lymphoid organs, employing mechanisms that are still mysterious, nTreg cells are able to suppress the activation of potentially self-reactive T cells. One way this may happen is by downregulating the expression of co-stimulatory molecules on antigen presenting cells. Suppression by nTregs appears to be antigen-specific: Only those T cells which recognize the same self antigen that the nTreg cell recognizes will be affected. Although there is a lot to be discovered about natural Tregs, it is clear that they play an important role in protecting us from autoimmune disease. Indeed, humans who have mutations that compromise the function of the Foxp3 protein suffer from aggressive autoimmune disease and die at an early age.

In the last lecture, I mentioned another type of regulatory T cell: the inducible regulatory T cell. Whereas the function of natural regulatory T cells is to provide protection against T cells which have the potential to react against <u>self</u> antigens and cause autoimmunity, the role of inducible regulatory T cells is quite different. Inducible regulatory cells are tasked with restraining the immune system to keep it from overreacting to the <u>foreign</u> antigens of invaders. Inducible and natural regulatory T cells also appear to differ in their mode of action. Natural regulatory T cells are thought to require direct, cell-to-cell contact to work their magic. In contrast, inducible regulatory T cells seem to function indirectly by producing cytokines which negatively regulate the immune system.

PERIPHERAL TOLERANCE

Of course, virgin T cells aren't perfect, and some do stray from the prescribed traffic pattern and venture out into the tissues. Indeed, potentially self-reactive T cells are found in the tissues of every normal human. There these "lawbreakers" may encounter self antigens that were too rare in the thymus to trigger deletion, but which are abundant enough in the tissues to activate these T cells. To deal with this situation, there is another level of protection against autoimmunity – peripheral tolerance.

Because of the two-key requirement for T cell activation, virgin T cells must not only encounter enough presented antigen to cluster their receptors, they must also receive co-stimulatory signals from the cell that is presenting the antigen. That's where activated antigen presenting cells come in. These special cells have lots of MHC molecules on their surface to present antigen, and they also express co-stimulatory molecules like B7. In contrast, "ordinary cells" like heart or kidney cells generally don't express high levels of MHC proteins or don't express co-stimulatory molecules, or both. As a result, a virgin T cell with receptors that recognize a kidney antigen could probably go right up to a kidney cell, and not be activated by it. In fact, it's even better than that. **When a T cell recognizes its cognate antigen presented on a cell, but does not receive the required co-stimulation, that T cell is "neutered." It looks like a T cell, but it can no longer perform. Immunologists say the cell is "anergized." In many cases, cells that are anergized eventually die, so peripheral tolerance induction can result in either anergy or death. Consequently, the requirement for the second, co-stimulatory "key" during T cell activation protects us against virgin T cells that venture outside their normal traffic pattern.**

TOLERANCE DUE TO ACTIVATION-INDUCED DEATH

Okay, so what if a T cell escapes deletion in the thymus, breaks the traffic laws, and ventures out into the tissues. And suppose that this T cell just happens to find its cognate antigen displayed by MHC molecules at a high enough density to crosslink its receptors on a cell that just happens to be able to provide the co-stimulation required to activate the T cell. What then? Well, all is not lost, because there is yet another "layer" of tolerance induction that can protect us in this unlikely situation.

In the last lecture, we discussed activation-induced cell death (AICD) as one way T cells are eliminated when an invader has been vanquished. This same mechanism also helps protect against virgin T cells that break the traffic rules and are activated by self antigens out in the tissues. T cells in this situation are stimulated over and over by the ever-present self antigens, and when this happens, the self-reactive T cells usually are eliminated by activation-induced cell death. It is as if the immune system senses that this continuous reactivation "ain't natural," and does away with the offending, self-reactive T cells.

In summary, induction of T cell tolerance is multilayered. No single mechanism of tolerance induction is 100% efficient, but because there are multiple mechanisms, autoimmune diseases are relatively rare. T cells with receptors that recognize antigens which are abundant in the secondary lymphoid organs usually are efficiently deleted in the thymus. Self antigens that are rare enough in the thymus to allow self-reactive T cells to escape deletion usually are also too rare to activate virgin T cells in the secondary lymphoid organs. Thus, because of their restricted traffic pattern, virgin T cells normally remain functionally ignorant of self antigens that are rare in the thymus. In addition, natural regulatory T cells in the secondary lymphoid organs are believed to provide additional protection, probably by interfering with the activation of potentially self-reactive T cells.

In those cases where virgin T cells do venture outside the blood–lymph–secondary lymphoid organ system, they generally encounter self antigens in a context that leads to anergy or death, not activation. Finally, those rare T cells that are activated by recognizing self antigens in the tissues usually die from chronic re-stimulation.

B CELL TOLERANCE

Immunologists once thought that it might not be necessary to delete B cells with receptors that recognize self antigens. The idea was that the T cells which were needed to help activate potentially self-reactive B cells would already have been killed or anergized, so that B cell tolerance would be "covered" by T cell tolerance. However, it now is clear that mechanisms also exist for tolerizing those B cells which have the potential to be self-reactive.

Most B cells are tolerized where they are born – in the bone marrow. This is the rough equivalent of thymic tolerance induction for T cells. After B cells mix and match gene segments to construct the genes for their receptors, they are "tested" to see if these receptors recognize self antigens that are present in the bone marrow. If its receptors do recognize a self antigen, a B cell is given another chance to rearrange its light chain gene and come up with new receptors that don't bind to a self antigen.

This process is called "receptor editing." Although the details of how receptor editing works are not yet understood, in mice at least 25% of all B cells take advantage of this "second chance." Nevertheless, even with this opportunity to try again to produce acceptable receptors, only about 10% of all B cells pass the tolerance test. The rest die in the bone marrow.

After testing, B cells with receptors that do not bind to self antigens which are abundant in the bone marrow are released to circulate with the blood and lymph. Of course, induction of B cell tolerance in the bone marrow has the same problems as T cell tolerance induction in the thymus: B cells which have receptors that recognize self antigens that are rare in the marrow can slip through the cracks. Fortunately, bone marrow contains mostly the same abundant self antigens that are found in the secondary lymphoid organs where virgin B cells will be activated. Consequently, self antigens that are too rare to efficiently delete B cells in the bone marrow usually are too rare to activate these B cells in the secondary lymphoid organs. So the traffic pattern of virgin B cells, which restricts them to circulating through the secondary lymphoid organs, helps protect them from encountering abundant self antigens that are not present in the bone marrow.

There are also mechanisms which can tolerize B cells that break these traffic laws. For example, virgin B cells that venture into the tissues can be anergized or deleted if they recognize their cognate antigen, but do not receive T cell help. Thus, B cells are subject to mechanisms which enforce self tolerance out in the tissues that are similar, but not identical, to those which tolerize T cells.

MAINTENANCE OF B CELL TOLERANCE IN GERMINAL CENTERS

In contrast to T cells, which are stuck with the same receptors they express when they are tested in the thymus, B cells have a chance, after they have been activated in the secondary lymphoid organs, to modify their receptors through somatic hypermutation. So you may be wondering whether B cells undergoing somatic hypermutation might end up with receptors that can recognize self antigens. If so, these B cells might produce antibodies that could cause autoimmune disease. Fortunately, it turns out that this usually doesn't happen, and the reasons are quite interesting.

B cells in germinal centers are very "fragile." Unless they receive "rescue" signals, they die by apoptosis. In this sense, germinal center B cells resemble the fragile T cells that are subject to MHC restriction and tolerance induction in the thymus. The signals required to rescue B cells from death in a germinal center are the same as those required to activate B cells in the first place: recognition of cognate antigen in a form that crosslinks BCRs, plus co-stimulatory signals from helper T cells. B cells seem to need these two types of rescue signals more or less continuously while they are in the germinal center. Now if a B cell hypermutates in a germinal center so that its receptors recognize a self antigen, it is very unlikely to find (and be rescued by) that self antigen advertised on follicular dendritic cells. After all, FDCs only display antigens that have been opsonized – and self antigens usually aren't opsonized.

So the first difficulty that potentially self-reactive B cells face in a germinal center is the lack of opsonized self antigen on follicular dendritic cells. But they have another problem – lack of co-stimulation – and the reason for this is even more interesting. After Th cells have been activated in the T cell zones of secondary lymphoid organs, they move to lymphoid follicles to give help to B cells. This help takes place during a "dance" in which the Th cell and the B cell stimulate each other. While dancing, the Th cell provides the CD40L needed to co-stimulate the B cell. In return, the activated B cell satisfies the helper cell's needs not only by supplying B7 co-stimulation, but also by using its class II MHC molecules to present fragments of its cognate antigen to the Th cell. The subtle, but important, point here is that for this mutual activation thing between a B cell and a T cell to work, these cells must be looking at parts of the same antigen. So if a B cell hypermutates so that its BCRs bind to, internalize, and present a self antigen, that new antigen will not be recognized by the "needy" Th cell's receptors. As a result, the B and T cells will not be able to cooperate to keep each other stimulated. They will have lost their "common interest." And because B cells require T cell help to survive in the germinal center, the interdependence of B and T cells keeps B cells "on track" as they undergo somatic hypermutation. So self tolerance is preserved during B cell hypermutation for two reasons: the lack of opsonized self antigen required for efficient BCR signaling, and the lack of germinal center Th cells which can provide help for B cells that recognize self antigen.

SUMMARY FIGURE

T cell tolerance is a multilayered process in which multiple levels of tolerance-inducing mechanisms insure that, for most humans, autoimmunity never happens.

T CELLS WHICH RECOGNIZE **ABUNDANT** SELF ANTIGENS IN THYMUS ARE ELIMINATED
CENTRAL TOLERANCE

VIRGIN T CELLS DON'T "SEE" ABUNDANT SELF ANTIGENS IN TISSUES BECAUSE OF RESTRICTED TRAFFIC PATTERN
TRAFFIC PATTERNS

ACTIVATION SUPPRESSED BY nTREGs
SECONDARY LYMPHOID ORGANS

VIRGIN T CELLS DIE OR ARE ANERGIZED IN TISSUES DUE TO LACK OF TCR CROSS-LINKING OR CO-STIMULATION
MISSING SIGNALS

T CELLS ARE DELETED DUE TO **CHRONIC** STIMULATION BY SELF ANTIGENS
ACTIVATION-INDUCED APOPTOSIS

THOUGHT QUESTIONS

1. Why is it important that T cells be tested to be sure they can recognize self MHC molecules? Wouldn't it be a lot simpler just to eliminate this exam?

2. For T cells being educated in the thymus, what is the functional definition of self (i.e., what do these T cells consider to be self peptides)?

3. What is the underlying difficulty in a T cell satisfying both the requirement for MHC restriction (positive selection)

and the requirement for tolerance of self (negative selection)?

4. Why are mechanisms needed that can tolerize T cells once they leave the thymus?

5. Explain why the traffic pattern of virgin T cells plays a role in maintaining tolerance of self.

6. Why is it important that B cells also be taught tolerance of self?

LECTURE 10

Immunological Memory

REVIEW

In the last lecture, we discussed one of the most important riddles in immunology: how can the same T cell receptor mediate positive selection (MHC restriction), negative selection (tolerance induction), and activation? The current thinking is that positive selection (survival) of T cells whose receptors recognize self MHC results from a relatively weak interaction between TCRs and MHC–self peptides displayed on cortical thymic epithelial cells. This "test" is intended to focus the attention of T cells on antigen presented by MHC molecules, insuring that recognition is restricted to presented antigen, not "native" antigen. Negative selection (death) of cells with TCRs that recognize self antigen in the thymus is induced by a strong interaction between TCRs and MHC–self peptides expressed on bone marrow-derived, thymic dendritic cells and/or medullary thymic epithelial cells. This "exam" is designed to eliminate T cells which might cause autoimmune disease. Finally, after they leave the thymus, T cells can be activated to defend us against disease through a strong interaction between their TCRs and MHC–peptides displayed by professional antigen presenting cells.

One important point here is that the interactions which lead to these three very different outcomes are between the TCR and MHC-peptides displayed by very different types of cells. These cells can be expected to express different adhesion molecules, different co-stimulatory molecules, and even different cytokines – so the result of each of these interactions probably depends, at least in part, on the cell type with which the T cell interacts. In addition, T cells may learn from experience: their internal "wiring" may change as they are educated and mature. Consequently, as T cells grow up, the same signals may be processed differently and may produce different outcomes.

Although the mechanisms involved are not completely understood, the end result of the thymic experience is that only about 3% of the T cells that enter the screening process will exit from the thymus. These lucky T cells have receptors which do not recognize peptides derived from self antigens that are relatively abundant in the thymus. Of course, many T cells that exit the thymus will have receptors which can recognize foreign peptides presented by MHC – that's the whole idea of this game. But some of the thymic graduates will have receptors that recognize relatively rare self antigens which are not abundant enough in the thymus to efficiently delete T cells. So although thymic (central) tolerance induction is pretty good, it isn't the whole story. To take care of T cells that slip through thymic screening, several forms of "remedial education" exist outside the thymus that back up thymic tolerance induction.

One way of dealing with T cells that escape deletion in the thymus is to restrict the trafficking of virgin T cells to blood, lymph, and secondary lymphoid organs. Most self antigens that are abundant in the secondary lymphoid organs, where T cells are activated, also are abundant in the thymus. Consequently, T cells that could be activated by these self antigens already will have been deleted in the thymus. On the other hand, self antigens that are not abundant enough in the thymus to efficiently delete T cells usually are present in secondary lymphoid organs at concentrations too low to activate potentially self-reactive T cells. Therefore, because of their restricted traffic pattern, most virgin T cells with TCRs that recognize rare self antigens remain functionally ignorant of their existence, simply because they don't encounter enough of these antigens during their travels.

REVIEW (continued)

Occasionally, relatively large quantities of self antigens, which are too rare in the thymus to cause the deletion of T cells, do make their way to secondary lymphoid organs where they might activate formerly ignorant, potentially self-reactive T cells. However, to deal with this situation, there are mechanisms which help enforce self tolerance in the secondary lymphoid organs. For example, during their thymic education, some CD4+ T cells – probably those with receptors that have relatively high affinity for self antigens presented by class II MHC molecules – are selected to become natural regulatory T cells. These cells travel to the secondary lymphoid organs where they somehow help tolerize T cells which might otherwise be activated by self antigen.

Of course, not all virgin T cells are law-abiding, and some will leave their normal circulation pattern and wind up in the tissues. To deal with these "law breakers," Mother Nature has a few more tricks up her sleeve. For T cells to be activated, they must recognize their cognate MHC–peptide combination at a high enough concentration to trigger activation. Fortunately, most cells in the tissues don't express high enough levels of MHC–peptide to activate naive T cells. In addition, to be activated, virgin T cells must receive co-stimulatory signals from the cell that presents the antigen. Antigen presenting cells specialize in providing this co-stimulation, but your everyday cells out in the tissues do not. To take advantage of this fact, T cells are programmed so that when they recognize their cognate antigen, but do not receive adequate co-stimulation, they are anergized (neutered) or killed. Thus, even if cells in the tissues happen to express enough MHC–self peptide complexes to adequately crosslink the receptors on lawbreaking T cells, they generally don't express the co-stimulatory molecules required to rescue these T cells from death or anergy. In addition, even in the rare event that T cells are activated by self antigen in the tissues, these T cells usually die when they are chronically re-stimulated by the ever-present self antigen.

Tolerance induction in B cells is also multilayered. T cells have a separate organ, the thymus, in which central tolerance is induced. In contrast, B cells with receptors that recognize abundant self antigens are eliminated where they are born – in the bone marrow. Virgin B cells mainly travel through the blood, lymph, and secondary lymphoid organs. So like T cells, the traffic pattern of naive B cells usually protects them from contact with abundant self antigens on which they were not tested during tolerance induction in the bone marrow. Naive B cells that wander out of the blood/lymph traffic pattern usually don't encounter sufficient self antigen in a form that can crosslink their BCRs. In addition, virgin B cells whose receptors are crosslinked by self antigen in tissues usually don't receive the co-stimulatory signals required for activation – and crosslinking without co-stimulation can anergize or kill B cells.

The picture you should have is that none of the mechanisms for tolerizing B and T cells is foolproof – they all are a little "leaky." However, because there are multiple layers of tolerance-inducing mechanisms to catch potentially self-reactive cells, the whole system works very well, and relatively few humans suffer from serious autoimmune disease.

One of the most important attributes of the immune system is that it remembers past encounters with attackers. Both the innate and the adaptive systems have memories, but the mechanisms these two systems use to remember are quite different.

INNATE MEMORY

The innate immune system has a "hard-wired" memory which is extremely important in defending us against everyday invaders. This memory is the result of millions of years of experience, during which the innate system slowly evolved pattern-recognition receptors that can detect the signatures of common invaders. These receptors (e.g., the Toll-like receptors we discussed in Lecture 4) detect molecular structures which are characteristic of broad classes of microbial pathogens, and which usually are indispensable for an invader's lifestyle. Because pattern-recognition receptors are standard equipment for cells of the innate system, this ancient memory allows an immediate and robust response to invaders that have been attacking humans for a very long time. And because innate memory evolved as humans evolved, all of us have the same innate memory.

ADAPTIVE MEMORY

Whereas the innate immune system uses hard-wired, pattern-recognition receptors to detect pathogens which also plagued our ancestors, **the adaptive immune system is set up to remember attackers we encounter during our lifetime.** Although B and T cells have a diverse collection of receptors that can recognize essentially any invader, there are relatively few naive B or T cells with receptors that can recognize any particular attacker – not enough to mount an immediate defense. So in practical terms, B and T cells really begin life with a blank memory. During an initial attack, pathogen-specific B and T cells proliferate to build up their numbers – a process that takes one or two weeks. Only then are memory B and T cells generated that are sufficiently numerous to defend against a subsequent attack by the same invader. The way this memory is achieved is somewhat different for B cells and T cells, so let's begin by examining B cell memory.

B cell memory

It is clear that antibodies can confer life-long immunity to infection. For example, in 1781, Swedish traders brought the measles virus to the isolated Faeroe Islands. In 1846, when another ship carrying sailors infected with measles visited the islands, people who were older than 64 years did not contract the disease – because they still had antibodies against the measles virus. Even the longest-lived antibodies (the IgG class) have a half-life of less than a month, so antibodies would have to be made continuously over a period of many years to provide this long-lasting protection.

When B cells are activated during the initial response to an invader, three kinds of B cells are generated. First, short-lived plasma B cells are produced in the lymphoid follicles of secondary lymphoid organs. These cells travel to the bone marrow or spleen and produce huge quantities of antibodies that are specific for the attacker. Although they only live for a few days, short-lived plasma B cells produce antibodies which are extremely important in protecting us against an enemy that the immune system has never encountered before.

In addition to short-lived plasma B cells, two types of memory B cells are produced in germinal centers during an invasion. Importantly, the generation of both types of memory cells requires T cell help. The first kind of memory B cell is the long-lived plasma cell. In contrast to short-lived plasma cells, which are generated rapidly after infection and which die after a few heroic days,

long-lived plasma cells take up residence in the bone marrow, and continuously produce more modest amounts of antibodies. It is the long-lived plasma cells which manufacture the IgG antibodies that can provide life-long immunity to subsequent infections. So together, short-lived and long-lived plasma B cells provide both immediate and long-term antibody protection against attacks.

The second type of memory B cell is the central memory B cell. These cells reside mainly in the secondary lymphoid organs, and their job is not to produce antibodies. Central memory B cells function as memory "stem cells" which slowly proliferate to maintain a pool of central memory B cells, and to replace those long-lived plasma cells which have died of old age. In addition, if another attack occurs, central memory cells can quickly produce more, short-lived plasma B cells.

This strategy, which involves three types of B cells, makes good sense. When an invader first attacks, antibodies need to be made quickly to tag invaders for destruction. That's what short-lived plasma B cells do. If, at a later time, the invader attacks again, it is important to already have invader-specific antibodies made and deployed throughout the body as an immediate defense. That's the job of long-lived plasma B cells. And between attacks, readiness is maintained by central memory B cells. These cells replenish supplies of long-lived plasma cells, and also stand ready to produce a burst of short-lived plasma B cells – cells that can rapidly manufacture large quantities of invader-specific antibodies to overwhelm the enemy.

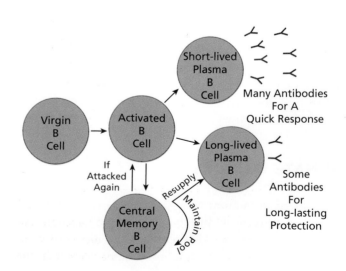

T cell memory

T cells also are able to remember a previous encounter with an invader. Indeed, it has been shown that memory T cells can persist for at least a decade. T cell memory is similar, but not identical, to B cell memory. **After naive T cells have been activated in response to an initial attack, and have proliferated to build up their numbers as much as 10 000-fold, many of them are given passports to travel out to the tissues to do battle with the enemy. These are the "effector" T cells. After the attack has been repulsed, most effector T cells die by apoptosis, but some of them, the "memory effector T cells," remain in the tissues. There they wait quietly for a subsequent attack. If that attack comes, they rapidly reactivate, proliferate a bit, and begin to destroy the invaders they remember.**

During an attack, some activated T cells do not travel out to the tissues to battle the invaders. They remain in the secondary lymphoid organs and the bone marrow. These are the "central memory T cells." During a subsequent attack, central memory T cells activate quickly, and after a brief period of proliferation, most mature into effector cells, which join the memory effector T cells at the battle scene. The rest of the central memory T cells remain in the secondary lymphoid organs and wait for another attack by the same invader.

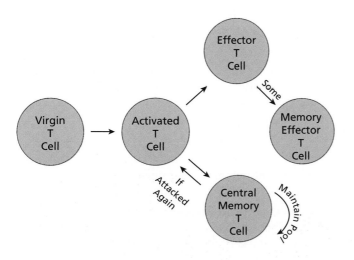

Properties of memory cells

The adaptive immune system remembers so well and reacts so powerfully during a subsequent infection that we usually don't even know we have been reinfected. There are a number of reasons why memory cells are better able to deal with a second attack than were the inexperienced B and T cells which responded to the original invasion. First, there are many more of them. Indeed, when we are attacked for the first time, there usually is only about one B or T cell in a million which can recognize that invader. In contrast, by the time the battle is over, the pool of pathogen-specific cells will have expanded so that roughly one in a thousand of all the B or T cells will recognize the attacker. Consequently, **the adaptive immune system's response to a subsequent attack is much more robust than the initial response – because there are so many more invader-specific cells "on duty."**

In addition to being more numerous than their inexperienced predecessors, **memory B and T cells are easier to activate.** The latest thinking is that during re-activation of memory cells, recognition of cognate antigen is required, but at least in some cases, co-stimulation is not essential. Now why would it be advantageous to have a system in which it is difficult to activate a B or T cell the first time, but relatively easier to reactivate it? Clearly, we want activation of virgin cells to be tightly controlled, because we only want to activate the adaptive immune system when there is a real threat. Consequently, a failsafe activation requirement for virgin B and T cells is important. On the other hand, once these cells have been through the stringent, two-key selection for primary activation, we want them to respond quickly to a subsequent attack by the same invader. So making it easier for them to be re-activated makes perfect sense.

There is a third reason why memory B cells are better defenders than are naive B cells: **memory B cells are "upgraded" versions of the original, virgin B cells.** These upgrades are of two types. First, **during the course of an attack, B cells gradually switch the class of antibody they make from the "compromise" antibody class, IgM, to one of the other classes (IgG, IgA, or IgE) which specializes in dealing with that particular kind of invader. This class switch is imprinted on the memory of the B cells that remain after an attack. As a result, memory B cells are able to produce the antibody class which is just right to protect against the invader they remember.**

Also, **during an attack, B cells use somatic hypermutation to fine-tune both their receptors and the antibodies they manufacture.** Hypermutation results in upgraded B cell receptors that can detect small amounts of foreign antigen early in an attack, allowing central memory B cells to be activated quickly during a subsequent infection. Moreover, because of hypermutation, long-lived plasma cells make upgraded antibodies that can bind more tightly to the invader.

Comparing B and T cell memories

B and T cell memories are similar in that both systems center around stem-cell-like central memory cells. These central memory cells reside in the secondary lymphoid organs, where they are strategically located to intercept invaders as they enter the body. In addition, memory B and T cells are more potent weapons than are naive cells because a larger fraction of them are specific for the invader they remember – and because they are easier to activate.

Other aspects of B cell and T cell memory, however, are different. In response to an invasion, B cells can fine-tune their receptors through somatic hypermutation. T cells cannot. Moreover, there is no T cell equivalent of the long-lived plasma B cell. Once we have been exposed to an invader, long-lived plasma B cells continue to produce protective antibodies, frequently for a lifetime. Consequently, the weapons made by B cells (the antibody molecules) continue to be deployed even after an invasion has been repulsed. This works well because antibodies are very specific and rather benign. Only when they tag an invader is the rest of the immune system alerted to take action. So if the invader they recognize doesn't come again, the pre-made antibodies do nothing and cause no trouble.

In contrast, activated T cells produce cytokines and other chemicals which are nonspecific and which can cause severe damage to normal tissues. As a result, it would be very dangerous to have T cells remain in action once an invasion has been repulsed. Consequently, instead of continuing to function after the enemy has been defeated, as long-lived plasma cells do, effector memory T cells go "dormant." If the attacker does not return, they cause no trouble. On the other hand, if an enemy again enters the tissues where effector memory T cells are "sleeping," these cells quickly reactivate and spring into action.

How B and T cell memory is maintained

One of the puzzles about adaptive memory is how it can be maintained for a lifetime, even if an invader has been eliminated from the body and never returns. Antibodies have life spans measured in days or weeks, long-lived plasma cells only survive for a few months, and memory effector T cells also have relatively short lives. Consequently, memory cells and antibodies must be continuously replenished to provide lasting memory.

It was first assumed that "remnants" of the initial infection (e.g., pieces of a virus or a bacterium) were retained in the secondary lymphoid organs, and that these antigens might re-stimulate central memory cells and cause them to proliferate slowly to replace long-lived plasma cells or effector memory T cells which died of old age. However, recent experiments have shown that although this type of re-stimulation does take place, memory actually can be sustained without any traces of the original infection being present. It is thought that certain cytokines trigger memory T cells to proliferate slowly, independent of their TCR specificity, and that memory B cells proliferate when their pattern recognition receptors or their BCRs are ligated weakly by self antigens. Nevertheless, more research is needed to fully understand how B and T cell memory is maintained once an invader has been vanquished.

INNATE VERSUS ADAPTIVE MEMORY

Although both innate and adaptive immune systems remember, it is important to understand how these memories differ. The innate memory is a static memory: it is not updatable – at least not on the time scale of a human lifetime. Although there may be slight genetic differences from human to human, all humans have essentially the same innate memory, which reflects the experience of the human race with common invaders that have been plaguing us for millions of years.

In contrast, the adaptive immune system has an expandable memory which can remember any invader to which we have been exposed, be it common or rare. Moreover, the adaptive immune system's memory is personal: each of us has a different adaptive memory, depending on the particular invaders we have encountered during our lifetime. In fact, even when two people have been attacked by the same microbe, their adaptive memories of that attack will be different – because the receptors on the collection of invader-specific B and T cells will differ from person to person. Indeed, because B and T cell receptors are made by a mix-and-match mechanism, no two humans will have the same adaptive memory.

THOUGHT QUESTIONS

1. What are the basic differences between innate system memory and adaptive system memory?

2. What properties of memory B and T cells make them better able to defend against a subsequent infection?

3. Explain how B cell memory protects us against invaders in both the near and distant future.

4. How does T cell memory protect us against invaders in the near future and beyond?

5. What are the differences between the strategies B and T memory cells use to be sure we are "covered" against a future invasion by the pathogen they remember? Why are these differences important?

6. So far, we have encountered three types of dendritic cells: antigen presenting DCs, follicular DCs, and thymic dendritic cells. As a way to review, explain the function of each of these cell types.

LECTURE 11

Vaccines

REVIEW

Both the innate and adaptive systems are able to remember past invaders. The innate immune system's memory is hard-wired, and depends on pattern-recognition receptors that have evolved over millions of years to identify common invaders. These receptors recognize signatures which are shared by classes of invaders (e.g., all bacteria that have LPS as a cell wall component), and focus on molecular structures that are not easily mutated. All humans have the same innate memory. In contrast, B and T cells of the adaptive immune system have "updatable" memories which can remember the individual invaders we have encountered during our lifetimes, both common and rare. Adaptive memory is "personal" in the sense that every person has a different adaptive memory.

T and B cell memories both require that central memory cells persist in the secondary lymphoid organs following an attack. Central memory T cells react quickly to a second attack by proliferating and maturing into effector T cells, which can travel to the site of the invasion, and destroy the enemy. Between attacks, central memory T cells proliferate slowly to maintain a pool of central memory T cells.

Central memory B cells also are produced during an attack. If we are invaded again by the same pathogen, central memory B cells quickly activate, proliferate, and most of them mature into plasma B cells – cells which can produce large quantities of pathogen-specific antibodies. Also remaining after a first attack are long-lived plasma B cells which reside in the bone marrow. These cells continuously produce moderate amounts of pathogen-specific antibodies, which give us immediate protection if we are attacked again. This pool of long-lived plasma cells is continually replenished by central memory cells, which proliferate slowly between invasions.

Memory B and T cells are better able to deal with a second attack because they are much more numerous than before the first invasion, and because they are more easily activated than are virgin B and T cells. Moreover, memory B cells have receptors that have been fine-tuned by somatic hypermutation, and memory B cells usually have class switched to produce the type of antibody molecule which is most appropriate for the invader they remember. As a result of these upgrades, memory B cells are more efficient at dealing with repeat offenders than were their virgin ancestors.

During many "natural" infections, memory B and T cells are generated which can provide protection against a subsequent attack. However, a natural infection can be quite devastating – even lethal. If there were some safe way to trick the immune system into thinking it had been attacked, and to get it to produce memory B and T cells that are appropriate to defend against the perceived attacker, then a person could be protected against a real (natural) infection. And that, of course, is what a vaccination does.

A vaccination is the immunological equivalent of the war games our armed forces use to prepare troops for battle. The goal of these "games" is to give soldiers as realistic a simulation of battle conditions as is possible without putting them in great danger. Likewise, a vaccination is intended to prepare the immune system for battle by giving the system as close a look at the real thing as is possible without exposing the vaccine recipient to undue risks. Consequently, the generals who plan the war games and the scientists who develop vaccines have a common aim: maximum realism with minimum danger.

Vaccines have been extremely useful in controlling infectious diseases. For example, before a diphtheria vaccine was available, the number of new cases of diphtheria in the United States reached over 350 000 per year. Now, as a result of widespread vaccination against diphtheria, usually fewer than five cases are reported annually.

GENERATING MEMORY HELPER T AND B CELLS

When we are first exposed to an invader, dendritic cells at the battle site ingest the attacker or fragments of the attacker, and travel to nearby lymph nodes. There they use class II MHC molecules to present peptides derived from the invader's proteins. If a helper T cell has receptors which recognize these peptides, it can be triggered to proliferate. Eventually, some of these helper T cells become memory cells which can help protect against a subsequent attack. So for memory helper T cells to be generated, all that is required is for dendritic cells to collect "debris" from the battle scene (e.g., viral coat proteins or part of a bacterial cell wall) and present peptides derived from this debris to helper T cells.

Likewise, when a B cell's receptors recognize an attacker or a fragment of an attacker which has been transported to the secondary lymphoid organs by the lymph or the blood, that B cell can be activated if it receives T cell help. After a period of proliferation, some of the resulting B cells will become memory cells to provide protection from future attacks by the same invader. So as with helper T cells, even a bit of battle debris is enough to activate a B cell and generate memory B cells. The important point here is that memory B and helper T cells can be produced efficiently even when no immune system cells have been infected by the attacker.

GENERATING MEMORY KILLER T CELLS

Memory killer T cells also can be produced during a microbial attack, but for this to happen, the microbe must infect an antigen presenting cell. For example, if a virus infects a dendritic cell, it will commandeer the cell's biosynthetic machinery to make viral proteins as part of its reproductive strategy. Some of these proteins will be chopped up into peptides and loaded onto class I MHC molecules. As a result, killer T cells whose receptors recognize the virus' peptides will be activated, and if assistance is available from helper T cells, memory killer T cells will be produced.

So the requirements for generating memory helper T and B cells are different from those for generating memory CTLs. **Memory helper T cells and B cells can be produced even when an invader does not infect an antigen presenting cell. In contrast, for memory killer T cells to be made, the attacker must infect an antigen presenting cell.**

As I mentioned in Lecture 4, under certain experimental conditions, antigen presenting cells can use class I MHC molecules to present antigens that are taken up from outside the cell. In this case, virus-specific CTLs can be generated even when the virus does not infect antigen presenting cells. This phenomenon is termed "cross-presentation." Currently, the rules that govern cross-presentation are not well understood, and it is not known how important cross-presentation actually is for the normal functioning of the human immune system. Indeed, no anti-viral vaccine has been devised that uses cross-presentation to generate protective CTL memory in humans. Of course, it is possible that cross-presentation may eventually be used to produce a vaccine. However, at this time the rule seems to be that for a vaccine to efficiently generate memory CTLs, antigen presenting cells must be infected. In this lecture, we'll stick to this rule.

STRATEGIES FOR VACCINE DEVELOPMENT

A number of different strategies have been employed to develop the vaccines currently used to protect against microbial infections. In addition, there are innovative, new approaches to vaccine design which are being tested. One important feature of a vaccination is that its efficacy does not depend on the recipient altering his level of hygiene or his lifestyle. Consequently, many believe that a vaccine against HIV-1 may be the best way to stop the spread of AIDS. Because this disease is such an important health issue, as we discuss different types of vaccines, we will ask whether any of them might be suitable to use as a vaccine that would protect against an HIV-1 infection. In the end, I think you will agree that designing a safe and effective AIDS vaccine is a difficult challenge.

A major obstacle to producing an effective AIDS vaccine is that it isn't certain which types of memory cells are needed. The results of trials with vaccines that only produce memory B cells and antibodies suggest that antibodies alone cannot protect against an HIV-1 infection. In contrast, individuals who are infected with HIV-1, but whose immune systems resist the virus for long periods of time, usually have inherited particular class I MHC molecules – suggesting that presentation of antigens to killer T cells is important for resistance. Consequently, **most immunologists believe that an effective AIDS vaccine must generate memory killer T cells.** Unfortunately, the production of memory CTLs requires that the agent used as a vaccine be capable of infecting antigen presenting cells – and this puts severe restrictions on the types of AIDS vaccines that might be safe to use.

Non-infectious vaccines

Many vaccines are designed not to infect the vaccine recipient. The Salk vaccine for polio is an example of such a "non-infectious" vaccine. To make his vaccine, Dr Salk treated polio virus with formaldehyde to "kill" the virus. Formaldehyde acts by gluing proteins together, and the result of this treatment is a virus that looks to the immune system very much like a live poliovirus, but which cannot infect cells because its proteins are non-functional. This treatment is the molecular equivalent of the parking police applying a "boot" to the wheel of a car. The car may look quite normal, but because the wheels can't turn, the vehicle is disabled. The common flu vaccine also is a killed virus vaccine, and a similar strategy has been used to make vaccines against disease-causing bacteria. For example, the typhoid vaccine and an effective pertussis (whooping cough) vaccine both are prepared from bacteria that have been grown in the lab and then treated with chemicals like formaldehyde.

Although the chemicals used to kill these microbes certainly will incapacitate most of them, the procedure is not guaranteed to be 100% effective, and some of them may survive. Now if a vaccine is intended to protect against a virus like influenza, which otherwise will infect a large fraction of the population, a few live viruses in the vaccine preparation is not a major concern – because without vaccination, many more people would contract the disease. In contrast, for adults in developed countries where blood

supplies are carefully screened, infection with HIV-1 is preventable, except in rare cases. Consequently, a vaccine that has even a small probability of causing the disease could not be used to vaccinate the general public.

Some bacteria produce proteins called toxins that actually cause the symptoms associated with the bacterial infection. In a few cases, these toxins have been used as non-infectious vaccines. To prepare such a vaccine, the toxin is purified, and treated with aluminum salts to produce a weakened form of the toxin called a toxoid. When injected into a recipient, the toxoid mobilizes B cells which produce antibodies that can bind to and inactivate the harmful toxin during a real attack. Vaccines made from diphtheria or tetanus toxins are examples of this type of non-infectious vaccine.

Non-infectious vaccines also have been prepared by using only certain parts of a pathogen. The idea here is to retain the portions that the immune system needs to see for protection, while discarding the parts that cause unpleasant or dangerous side effects. An "acellular" vaccine for pertussis is made in this way. The original pertussis vaccine was prepared from whole, killed pertussis bacteria, and about half of the infants inoculated with that vaccine had an adverse reaction to it. Fortunately, almost all these side effects were mild when compared with the life-threatening possibility of contracting whooping cough. The acellular vaccine is prepared by growing the pertussis bacteria in culture and then purifying several of the bacterial proteins away from the rest of the bacterial components. The acellular vaccine is now the vaccine of choice, because it has a much lower rate of adverse reactions than the original pertussis vaccine, yet is equally effective in preventing whooping cough.

Viral proteins produced by genetic engineering also can be used as non-infectious, "subunit" vaccines. The highly effective vaccines against hepatitis B virus and the human papilloma virus both are made in this way. Because only one or a few "synthetic" viral proteins are used to make a subunit vaccine, there is no possibility of infection with the microbe itself (e.g., the hepatitis B virus).

A potential drawback of all non-infectious vaccines is that although they will generate memory helper T cells and B cells (which can make protective antibodies), memory killer T cells will not be made – because antigen presenting cells will not be infected. Of course, many pathogens (e.g., extracellular bacteria) do not infect human cells at all. Consequently, the lack of memory CTLs (which kill infected cells) is not an issue in designing vaccines for these microbes. Also, antibodies produced by memory B cells are sufficient to protect against many pathogens, including some pathogens which do infect human cells. For example, poliovirus and hepatitis B virus infect human cells. Nevertheless, the non-infectious Salk poliovirus vaccine and the hepatitis B virus subunit vaccine both work very well even though neither vaccine generates memory killer T cells. In contrast, killed virus vaccines were unable to protect against either the measles or the mumps virus. So whether memory CTLs are required for protection depends on the particular microbe and its lifestyle.

Attenuated vaccines

Another strategy for producing a vaccine is to use a weak-ened or "attenuated" form of the microbe. Virologists noticed that when a virus is grown in the laboratory in a cell type which is not its normal host, the virus sometimes accumulates mutations which weaken it. The Sabin polio vaccine, for example, was made by growing poliovirus, which normally reproduces in human nerve cells, in monkey kidney cells. This strategy resulted in poliovi-ruses which were still infectious, but which were so weak that they could not cause the disease in healthy individu-als. The vaccines for measles, rubella, and mumps, which most children in the United States now receive, are atten-uated virus vaccines.

An attenuated vaccine can be tested on animals to get a general idea of whether the attenuation procedure has worked. However, to be sure a crippled microbe can stimulate the production of memory cells, yet not cause disease, it must be tested on humans – usually volunteers who expect to be at risk for contracting the disease. In this regard, it is interesting to note that by the time Dr Sabin was ready to test his vaccine, most people in our country had already received the Salk polio vaccine. So Dr Sabin took his vaccine to Russia and tested it there. This was at the height of the Cold War, but polio was such a dreaded disease that the Russians were delighted to be "guinea pigs" for Dr Sabin's vaccine.

One important feature of attenuated virus vaccines is that they can produce memory killer T cells. This is because the crippled virus can infect antigen presenting cells and stimulate the production of CTLs before the immune system has had a chance to destroy the weak-ened invaders. However, because an attenuated vaccine contains a microbe that is infectious, there are safety issues. When a person has recently been vaccinated with an attenuated virus vaccine, he may produce enough virus to infect some of the people with whom he comes in contact. This can be an advantage if those people are healthy, because it "spreads the immunity around." However, a person whose immune system is weakened (e.g., because of chemotherapy for cancer) may not be able to subdue the attenuated virus. After all, the attenu-ated microbe in the vaccine isn't dead. It's just weak. So for those who are immunosuppressed, this type of gra-tuitous vaccination can have serious consequences.

A second potential safety issue with an attenuated virus vaccine is that before the recipient's immune system subdues the weakened virus, the virus may mutate, and these mutations may restore the strength of the virus. Although this is not a very likely scenario, some healthy people who received the Sabin attenuated vaccine have contracted polio because the weakened virus mutated and regained its ability to cause disease.

Carrier vaccines

One new strategy for vaccine preparation uses genetic engineering to introduce a single gene from a pathogenic microbe into a virus that doesn't cause disease. This engineered virus can then be employed as a "Trojan horse" to carry the gene of the pathogenic microbe into human cells. The idea here is that if the carrier infects the vaccine recipient's antigen presenting cells, these cells will produce the pathogenic microbe's protein as well as the carrier's own proteins. As a result, vaccination with a carrier vaccine should generate memory killer T cells that can protect against a future attack by the real pathogen. Importantly, there is no chance that this vaccine will cause the disease it is designed to protect against – because only one of the pathogen's many genes is "carried" by the vaccine.

It might seem that this approach would be perfect to use to prepare an AIDS vaccine, and vaccines of this type are now being tested. Most recently, a vaccine trial in Thailand used a canarypox virus (a cousin of Jenner's cowpox virus) as a Trojan horse to carry in several genes for HIV-1 proteins. This carrier virus vaccination was then "boosted" by vaccinating the same individuals with a subunit vaccine containing a synthetic version of one of the same HIV-1 proteins produced by the carrier virus. The people receiving these vaccinations, and a roughly equal number of individuals who received a placebo vac-cination, were followed for a period of three years to determine how many in each group subsequently became infected with the AIDS virus as a result of risky sexual behavior. Although the authors claimed that the trial "showed a significant, though modest, reduction in the rate of HIV-1 infection," the data is not very convincing. During the study period, 56 people who received the authentic vaccine became infected, whereas 76 members of the group which received the sham vaccine became infected. These are very small numbers on which to base a meaningful conclusion. Moreover, HIV-specific T cells could only be detected in about 17% of the people who received the vaccine. Finally, when the people who became infected were tested, there was no significant difference in the amount of virus in the blood of members of the two groups. This would suggest that the vaccination had little effect on the ability of infected individuals to resist the viral infection – not what you would expect from a vaccine.

WILL THERE BE AN AIDS VACCINE?

Most immunologists believe that to be effective, an AIDS vaccine must generate memory killer T cells. If true, non-infectious vaccines, which have been used to protect against many other pathogens, will be of little use against HIV-1. In principle, a weakened form of the AIDS virus could be used as a vaccine that would produce memory CTLs. However, because the AIDS virus has an extremely high mutation rate, there is great concern that an attenuated form of HIV-1 might mutate to become lethal again. Consequently, it is very unlikely that a vaccine which uses an attenuated version of the AIDS virus could ever be used to vaccinate the general population. A carrier vaccine could generate memory killer T cells without putting the vaccine recipient at risk for a real AIDS virus infection. So far, however, this strategy has not yielded a vaccine powerful enough to elicit an immune response against HIV-1 that is protective.

Even if a safe vaccine could be devised which would produce HIV-1-specific CTLs, the high mutation rate of the AIDS virus makes it an elusive target. On average, each AIDS virus produced by an infected cell differs from the original infecting virus by at least one mutation.

Consequently, the body of someone infected with HIV-1 contains not just "the" AIDS virus, but a huge collection of slightly different, HIV-1 strains. As a result, the memory cells produced by a vaccination might protect very well against the particular strain of HIV-1 used to prepare the vaccine, yet be totally useless against other mutant versions of the virus present in a real infection. Indeed, the virus' ability to mutate rapidly may prove to be the most difficult problem of all to solve in making an effective AIDS vaccine.

Despite all these difficulties, immunologists are working hard to produce an AIDS vaccine that can be used to protect the public – because such a vaccine is viewed as the current best hope for controlling the spread of the AIDS virus. Recently, antibodies have been discovered in rare AIDS patients which can neutralize many different HIV-1 variants. If a vaccine could be made which would elicit these "broadly neutralizing" antibodies in healthy individuals, it might be able to protect them from infection, at least by many of the common HIV-1 strains. And, as we have discussed, it should be much easier to make a safe vaccine that produces protective antibodies than one which gives rise to HIV-1-specific killer T cells. Nevertheless, it may turn out that antibodies are not enough, and that virus-specific CTLs may be required for protection.

It is important to note, however, that HIV-1 is not the only microbe for which there is no effective vaccine. Roughly two million people die every year from malaria, yet there is no vaccine that has been shown to be protective against this disease. Likewise, immunologists have not been able to devise an effective vaccine against tuberculosis, a bacterial infection which kills about three million people each year. And roughly one third of all the people on earth are infected with herpes simplex virus, yet a herpes vaccine does not exist. Indeed, it is the hope of many that in trying to develop an AIDS vaccine, immunologists will discover new strategies that will make it possible to produce vaccines which will protect against some of these other pathogens for which vaccines currently are not available.

THOUGHT QUESTIONS

1. Compare the advantages and disadvantages of killed virus vaccines and attenuated virus vaccines.

2. What are the major obstacles to producing an AIDS vaccine for the general public?

LECTURE 12

The Immune System Gone Wrong

REVIEW

Vaccinations take advantage of the ability of B and T cells to remember invaders we have previously encountered. By introducing the immune system to a "safe" version of a microbe, vaccination prepares these adaptable weapons to respond more rapidly and more powerfully if a real attack occurs at some future time. The production of memory B and helper T cells does not require that an antigen presenting cell be infected, so a "non-infectious" vaccine made from a dead virus or even a single viral protein can be used to produce a vaccine that will elicit protective antibodies.

Designing a vaccine that will produce memory killer T cells is more difficult, because, so far, the only way to do this efficiently is with a vaccine that can infect antigen presenting cells. Most immunologists believe that to protect against HIV-1, a vaccine will need to elicit a strong CTL memory. However, an AIDS vaccine intended for use by the general public must have no possibility of causing the disease, and this places severe constraints on the types of HIV-1 vaccines that would be safe to use. It is possible that a carrier virus vaccine might produce a robust killer T cell memory, yet be safe for general use. Nevertheless, this approach has not yet yielded a generally useful AIDS vaccine.

Thus far, we have focused on the good that the immune system does in protecting us from infection. Occasionally, however, the immune system "goes wrong" – sometimes with devastating consequences. In this lecture we will examine several situations in which the immune system plays a major role in producing the damaging effects (the pathology) of a disease.

PATHOLOGICAL CONDITIONS CAUSED BY A NORMAL IMMUNE RESPONSE

Tuberculosis is an example of a disease in which the pathology is the unintended consequence of normal immune system function. Tuberculosis is usually contracted by inhaling microdroplets containing the TB bacterium (*Mycobacterium tuberculosis*) that are generated by the cough of an infected individual. When these bacteria are taken into the lungs, they are confronted by macrophages, which are stationed there to intercept invaders that enter via the respiratory tract. A macrophage first engulfs an invader in a phagosome. This vesicle is then taken inside the macrophage where it fuses with a lysosome that contains powerful chemicals which can destroy most bacteria.

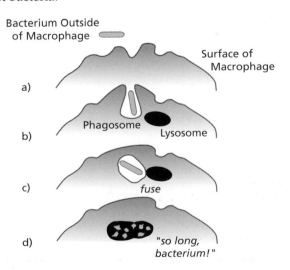

Unfortunately, in the case of the tuberculosis bacterium, the macrophage bites off more than it can chew, because the devious TB bacterium is able to modify the surface of the phagosome so that it does not fuse with the lysosome. Within the phagosome, the bacterium is safe, and it has easy access to all the nutrients it needs to grow and multiply. Indeed, it is ironic that a TB bacterium happily spends most of its life inside a macrophage – a defender that is supposed to deal harshly with bacterial attackers.

Eventually, many newly minted TB bacteria burst out of the macrophage, killing it. These bacteria then go on to infect other macrophages in the area. As a macrophage dies by necrosis, the contents of its lysosomes are released into the tissues of the lungs. This damages the lungs, and initiates an inflammatory reaction which recruits other immune system cells to the battle site, causing even more tissue damage.

The struggle between macrophages and TB bacteria results in the production of battle cytokines that can hyperactivate macrophages in the lungs. Once hyperactivated, the killing power of its weapons increases, so a macrophage can better deal with TB bacteria. Unfortunately, some of the chemicals given off by hyperactivated macrophages cause additional damage to the tissues of the lungs.

Macrophages and the cells they recruit sometimes win this battle and eliminate the invading bacteria or at least contain them. In other cases, it's a fight to a draw, and a state of chronic inflammation results in which the bacteria are kept in check, but macrophages continue to be killed, and the lungs continue to be damaged by the inflammatory reaction. So in a TB infection, the pathology of the disease results from macrophages doing exactly what they are supposed to do – engulf invaders and summon additional immune system cells to help fight the battle.

Sepsis is another disease caused by the immune system trying to do the right thing. Every year, about 250 000 Americans die from sepsis. One important feature of the immune response is that it usually is "local." Under normal conditions, our bodies must be defended against numerous small attacks which can come at any point along the boundaries that separate our bodies from the outside world. For this reason, our defense system is set up to provide rapid and vigorous responses to these attacks. The aim of this potent, local defense is to subdue the enemy quickly before it has a chance to "dig in" and establish its own base of operations. There can be a downside, however, to such a powerful defense: if there is an invasion which is <u>not</u> local, one that affects the whole body, the summation of the potent local immune defenses can actually be life-threatening. Sepsis is a rather generic term that describes the symptoms which can result from such a systemic infection.

Sepsis usually is caused by bacteria that enter the blood stream when the physical barriers which are our first line of defense are breached. For sepsis to occur in a healthy individual, a large number of bacteria must be introduced into the circulation. This can occur, for example, as a result of bacterial escape from an abscess or other formerly localized infection. In patients with a suppressed immune system (e.g., during chemotherapy for cancer), much smaller quantities of bacteria are required.

Although both Gram-negative and Gram-positive bacteria can cause sepsis, the classic culprits are Gram-negative bacteria like *E. coli* which have lipopolysaccharide (LPS) as a component of their cell walls. These bacteria also shed this molecule into their surroundings, and LPS is a potent danger signal that can activate macrophages and NK cells. These two cells then cooperate in a positive feedback loop that increases their activation states. Normally, this positive feedback loop amplifies the immune response, so that the innate system can respond quickly and strongly to a localized infection. However, in a "full-body" infection in which bacteria carried by the blood enter tissues everywhere, this amplified response can get out of hand. TNF secreted by activated macrophages can cause blood vessels to become "leaky," so that fluid escapes from the vessels into the surrounding tissues. In extreme cases, the decrease in blood volume due to system-wide leakage can cause a drop in blood pressure that results in shock (septic shock) and heart failure. So sepsis and septic shock can result when positive feedback loops, which normally allow the innate immune system to react strongly and quickly, cause an over-reaction to a system-wide infection.

DISEASES CAUSED BY DEFECTS IN IMMUNE REGULATION

Roughly a quarter of the US population suffers from allergies to common environmental antigens (allergens) that either are inhaled or ingested. Hay fever and asthma are the two most common allergic diseases of the respiratory tract. Hay fever is caused by proteins that are derived from mold spores or plant pollens. These allergens are present in the outside air, usually at certain times of the year. In contrast, the allergens that cause asthma are mostly found indoors. Dust mites, cockroaches, rodents, and household pets are major sources of these allergy-causing proteins. In addition to allergies caused by allergens in the air we breathe, the food we eat can also cause allergies.

The immune systems of non-allergic people respond weakly to these allergens, and produce mainly antibodies of the IgG class. In striking contrast, allergic individuals (called "atopic" individuals) produce large quantities of IgE antibodies. Indeed, the concentration of IgE antibodies in the blood of those with allergies can be 1000- to 10 000-fold higher than in the blood of non-atopic people! **It is the overproduction of IgE antibodies in response to otherwise innocuous environmental antigens that causes allergies.**

In Lecture 3, we discussed the interaction of IgE antibodies with white blood cells called mast cells. Because mast cell degranulation is a central event in many allergic reactions, let's take a moment to review this concept. When atopic individuals first are exposed to an allergen (e.g., pollen) they produce large amounts of IgE antibodies which recognize that allergen. Mast cells have receptors on their surface that can bind to the Fc region of IgE antibodies, so that after the initial exposure, mast cells will have large numbers of these allergen-specific IgE molecules attached to their surface. Allergens are small proteins with a repeating structure to which many IgE antibodies can bind close together. So on a second or subsequent exposure, an allergen can crosslink the IgE molecules on the mast cell surface, dragging the mast cell's Fc receptors together. This clustering of Fc receptors tells mast cells to "degranulate": to release their granules, which normally are stored safely inside the mast cells, into the tissues in which they reside. Mast cell granules contain histamine and other powerful chemicals and enzymes that can cause the symptoms with which atopic individuals are intimately familiar.

Interestingly, although IgE antibodies only live for about a day in the blood, once they are attached to mast cells, they have a half-life of several weeks. This means that mast cells can stay "armed" and ready to degranulate for an extended period after exposure to an allergen.

Allergic reactions generally have two phases: immediate and delayed. The immediate reaction to an allergen is the work of mast cells, which are stationed out in the tissues, and basophils, another granule-containing white blood cell, which can be recruited from the blood by signals given off by mast cells responding to an allergen. Like mast cells, basophils have receptors for IgE antibodies, and crosslinking of these receptors can lead to basophil degranulation.

Although mast cells and basophils are responsible for the immediate reaction to an allergen, a third, granule-containing white blood cell, the eosinophil, is the prominent player in chronic allergic reactions (e.g., in asthma). Before an "attack" by an allergen, there are relatively few eosinophils present in the tissues or circulating in the blood. However, once an allergic reaction has begun, helper T cells secrete cytokines such as IL-5 which can recruit many more eosinophils from the bone marrow. These eosinophils can then add their "weight" to the allergic reaction. Because eosinophils must be mobilized from the marrow, their contribution is delayed relative to that of mast cells and basophils, which can respond almost immediately.

Of course, mast cells, basophils, and eosinophils were not invented by Mother Nature just to annoy allergic people. These cells, with their ability to degranulate "on command," provide a defense against parasites (e.g., worms) that are too large to be phagocytosed by professional phagocytes. In a sense, IgE antibodies act as a "guidance system" for these cells, targeting their weapons to the enemy. For example, by discharging their destructive chemicals directly onto the skin (tegument) of a parasite to which IgE antibodies have bound, eosinophils can destroy these massive creatures.

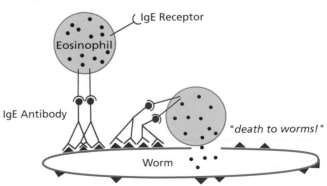

What makes this defense so elegant is that in response to a parasitic infection, parasite-specific IgE antibodies are made and mast cells, basophils, and eosinophils are armed – but nothing happens unless these armed cells come in contact with a parasite that can cluster their IgE receptors. Consequently, you don't get uncontrolled degranulation, wreaking havoc throughout your body. Rather, the IgE guidance system allows these cells to zero in on parasites, causing relatively little collateral damage to our tissues.

Why do some people have allergies?

It is clear that IgE antibodies are the bad guys in allergic reactions, but what determines whether a person will make IgE or IgG antibodies in response to an allergen? You remember from Lecture 6 that helper T cells can be "instructed" by the environment in which they are stimulated to secrete various cytokine subsets (e.g., Th1, Th2, or Th17). And the cytokines given off by these T cells can then influence B cells undergoing class switching to produce IgA, IgG, or IgE antibodies. For example, a germinal center that is populated with Th1 cells usually will produce B cells that make IgG antibodies, because Th1 cells secrete IFN-γ, which drives the IgG class switch. In contrast, B cells tend to change to IgE production if they class switch in germinal centers that contain Th2 cells which secrete IL-4 and IL-5. Consequently, **the decision to produce either IgG or IgE antibodies in response to an allergen will depend heavily on the type of helper T cells present in the secondary lymphoid organ which happens to intercept the allergen.** Indeed, helper T cells from allergic individuals show a much stronger bias toward the Th2 type than do Th cells from non-atopic people.

So atopic individuals produce IgE antibodies because their allergen-specific helper T cells tend to be of the Th2 type. But how do they get that way? The answer to this question is not known for certain, but many immunologists believe that a bias toward Th2-type helper T cells can be established early in childhood, and in some cases, even before birth. Here's how this is thought to work.

A fetus inherits roughly half of its genetic material from its mother and half from its father. As a result, the fetus is really a "transplant" that expresses many paternal antigens to which the mother's immune system is not tolerant. Since the placenta is the interface between the mother and the fetus, measures must be taken to avoid having maternal CTLs and NK cells attack the placenta because it expresses these paternal antigens. The Th1 subset of

helper cells secretes TNF, which helps activate NK cells, and IL-2, which causes NK cells and CTLs to proliferate. So it would be advantageous for the survival of the fetus to bias maternal Th cells away from the Th1 cytokine profile. Indeed, cells of the placenta produce relatively large amounts of IL-4, which influences maternal helper T cells to become Th2 cells. Importantly, these same placental cytokines also have a strong influence on <u>fetal</u> helper T cells. As a result, most humans are born with helper T cells that are strongly biased toward making Th2 cytokines.

Obviously this bias does not last a lifetime, and eventually most people end up with a more balanced population of Th1 and Th2 cells. One event that probably helps establish this balance is infection at an early age with microbes (e.g., viruses or bacteria) that normally elicit a Th1 response. Indeed, it is suspected that early microbial infections may be important in "reprogramming" the immune response so that a Th1 response to allergens results. Immunologists hypothesize that if a microbial infection strongly "deviates" the immune response of a young child toward a Th1 type at the same time that the child encounters an allergen (say, a dust mite protein), the Th response to that allergen also will be deviated toward the Th1 type. Once this deviation takes place, feedback mechanisms tend to lock in the Th1 response, and memory T cells will be generated that remember not only the allergen, but also their Th1 response to it. Once a large number of biased memory cells is built up, it is difficult to reverse this bias, so early exposure to infectious diseases may be critical in establishing a normal response to environmental allergens.

The idea that childhood microbial infections or early exposure to allergens might be important in biasing our immune systems toward producing Th1 helper T cells in response to environmental allergens is called the "hygiene hypothesis." Indeed, in Western countries, where improved personal hygiene has led to a decrease in childhood infections, and where exposure to certain allergens early in life is less frequent, the incidence of allergies to environmental allergens has increased dramatically. Some of the best data in support of the hygiene hypothesis comes from studies of families living on traditional farms. In fact, children in rural areas who grow up on farms have a significantly lower incidence of asthma and hay fever than do children from rural areas who do not live on a farm. This effect is even more pronounced if their mothers come in contact with multiple animal species and animal feed (such as hay and grain) during their pregnancy. Interestingly, the timing of exposure to animals and their feed seems to be important, with the greatest protection being observed for children who live on a farm during the first few years of their life. In this regard, it is important to note that living on a farm is not "unusual" as far as the human immune system is concerned. After all, until recently, many of our ancestors lived in close contact with farm animals, and it is likely that the immune system evolved to function best – at least in terms of allergies – in that setting.

It also has been proposed that regulatory T cells may help bias the immune system away from the production of IgE antibodies in response to environmental allergens. Helper T cells out in the tissues can be induced to become regulatory T cells (iTregs). Consequently, one could argue that if a person is routinely exposed to environmental allergens, some of his CD4$^+$ T cells may be induced to become regulatory T cells, which could suppress the immune response to these allergens. Indeed, inducible regulatory T cells produce IL-10 and TGFβ – cytokines which are known to bias antibody production away from IgE and toward IgG or IgA. Moreover, in individuals who are not atopic, regulatory T cells represent the majority of CD4$^+$ T cells that are specific for common environmental allergens. Although the idea that the induction of allergen-specific regulatory T cells might protect us from allergic reactions makes some sense, more research is required to validate this hypothesis.

Heredity

In addition to environmental factors (e.g., early exposure to infectious diseases or environmental allergens), heredity clearly plays a large part in susceptibility to allergies. For example, if one identical twin suffers from allergies, the probability is about 50% that the second twin will also be atopic. Immunologists have noticed that people who are allergic to certain allergens are more likely to have inherited particular class II MHC genes than are non-atopic people, suggesting that these MHC molecules may be especially efficient at presenting allergens. In addition, some atopic individuals produce mutant forms of the IgE receptor. It is hypothesized that these mutant receptors send an unusually strong signal when crosslinked, resulting in secretion of abnormally high levels of IL-4 by mast cells, and favoring the production of IgE antibodies. Mutations have even been detected in the regulatory (promoter) region of the IL-4 gene of some atopic individuals, and these mutations might increase the amount of IL-4 produced. Unfortunately, genes that confer susceptibility to allergies have been difficult to identify, because there seem to be many of them, and because they differ from atopic individual to atopic individual.

The best current synthesis of this information is that **the immunological basis for allergies is a defect in immune regulation in which allergen-specific helper T cells are strongly polarized toward a Th2 cytokine profile, resulting in the production of allergen-specific IgE antibodies. The genes a person inherits can make him more or less susceptible to allergies, and exposure to environmental factors such as microbial infections may influence whether susceptible individuals become atopic.**

Treatments for allergies

Although not a cure, treatment with glucocorticoid steroids can decrease allergy symptoms by blocking cytokine production by helper T cells. As a result, fewer B cells are activated (because they do not get the help they need), and the total number of antibodies made is reduced. Steroids, however, are not specific for allergies, and steroid treatment decreases the number of activated B cells of all kinds. Consequently, taking glucocorticoid steroids for extended periods can result in increased susceptibility to infectious diseases.

Recently, immunologists have produced antibodies (Omalizumab) which can grasp the Fc region of IgE antibodies and block the binding of these antibodies to mast cells. In human trials, these blocking antibodies relieved allergic symptoms and decreased the severity of asthma attacks. This treatment has now been approved for use in the United States, and it appears to be safe and effective – especially in severe cases.

So far, only one approach, "specific immunotherapy," has been successful in <u>curing</u> allergies. This treatment involves the injection of gradually increasing doses of crude extracts of allergens until a maintenance dose is achieved. Then, after several years of regular injections, some patients become tolerant to the allergen (or allergens) in the extract. Somehow, these injections encourage allergen-specific B cells to switch their antibody class from IgE to one of the other antibody classes. Indeed, during specific immunotherapy, the ratio of IgG to IgE antibodies specific for the allergen being administered can increase 10- to 100-fold. Unfortunately, the mechanism by which this immune deviation is achieved is not well understood, although the latest thinking is that repeated injections of allergen extracts may generate inducible regulatory T cells that produce cytokines which suppress IgE antibody production. Interestingly, this view is supported by the finding that beekeepers, who receive repetitive doses of bee venom (because they are stung frequently), do not suffer from severe allergic reactions, and have elevated levels of IL-10 – a cytokine produced by inducible regulatory T cells.

AUTOIMMUNE DISEASE

Rather than expend a huge amount of biological "energy" on a foolproof system in which every B and T cell is carefully checked for tolerance of self, Mother Nature evolved a multilayered system in which each layer includes mechanisms that should weed out most self-reactive cells, with lower layers catching cells that slip through tolerance induction in the layers above. This strategy works very well, but occasionally "mistakes are made" and instead of defending us against foreign invaders, the weapons of our immune system are turned back on us. **Autoimmune disease results when a breakdown in the mechanisms meant to preserve tolerance of self is severe enough to cause a pathological condition.** Roughly 5% of Americans suffer from some form of autoimmune disease.

Some cases of autoimmunity result from genetic defects. For example, most autoimmune diseases are chronic disorders that involve repeated stimulation of self-reactive lymphocytes. In normal people, this is controlled by activation-induced cell death in which chronically stimulated T cells are eliminated when Fas proteins on their surface are ligated. Humans with genetic defects in either the Fas or the Fas ligand proteins lack this layer of tolerance protection, and their T cells refuse to die when chronically stimulated by self antigens. The resulting diseases, **autoimmune lymphoproliferative syndrome** and **Canale–Smith syndrome**, have, as their pathological consequences, massive swelling of lymph nodes, production of antibodies that recognize self antigens, and the accumulation of large numbers of T cells in the secondary lymphoid organs.

Although some autoimmune disorders are due to genetic defects, **the majority of autoimmune diseases occur when the layers of tolerance-inducing mechanisms fail to eliminate self-reactive cells in genetically normal individuals.** In fact, you could argue that the potential for autoimmune disease is the price we must pay for having B and T cell receptors which are so diverse that they can recognize essentially any invader.

The latest thinking is that for autoimmunity to occur, at least three conditions must be met. First, an individual must express MHC molecules that efficiently present a peptide derived from the target self antigen. This means that the MHC molecules you inherit can play a major role in determining your susceptibility to autoimmune disease. For example, only about 0.2% of the US population suffers from juvenile diabetes, yet for Caucasian Americans who inherit two particular types of class II MHC genes, the probability of contracting this autoimmune disease is increased about twenty-fold.

The second requirement for autoimmunity is that the afflicted person must produce T and, in some cases, B cells which have receptors that recognize a self antigen. Because TCRs and BCRs are made by a mix-and-match strategy, the repertoire of receptors that one individual expresses will be different from that of every other individual, and will change with time as lymphocytes die and are replaced. Even the collections of TCRs and BCRs expressed by identical twins will be different. Therefore, it is largely by chance that a person will produce lymphocytes whose receptors recognize a particular self antigen.

So **for autoimmune disease to occur, a person must have MHC molecules that can present a self antigen as well as lymphocytes with receptors that can recognize the self antigen – but this is not enough. There also must be environmental factors that lead to the breakdown of the tolerance mechanisms which are designed to eliminate self-reactive lymphocytes.** For years, physicians have noticed that autoimmune diseases frequently follow bacterial or viral infections, and immunologists believe that microbial attack may be one of the key environmental factors that triggers autoimmune disease. Now clearly, a viral or bacterial infection cannot be the whole story, because for most people, these infections do not result in autoimmunity. However, in conjunction with a genetic predisposition (e.g., type of MHC molecules inherited) and lymphocytes with potentially self-reactive receptors, a microbial infection may be the "last straw" that leads to autoimmune disease.

Molecular mimicry

Immunologists' current favorite hypothesis to explain why infections might lead to the breakdown of self tolerance is called "molecular mimicry." Here's how this is thought to work.

Lymphocytes have BCRs or TCRs that recognize their cognate antigen. It turns out, however, that this is almost never a single antigen. Just as one MHC molecule can present a large number of peptides which have the same overall characteristics (length, binding motif, etc.), a TCR or a BCR usually can recognize ("cross-react with") several different antigens. Generally, a TCR or BCR will have a high affinity for one or a few of these cognate antigens, and relatively lower affinities for the others.

During a microbial invasion, lymphocytes whose receptors recognize microbial antigens will be activated. The molecular mimicry hypothesis holds that sometimes these receptors also recognize a self antigen, and if they do, an autoimmune response to that self antigen may result. It is presumed that before the microbial infection, these potentially self-reactive lymphocytes had not been activated either because the affinity of their receptors for the self antigen was too low to trigger activation, or because the restricted traffic patterns of virgin lymphocytes never brought them into contact with the self antigen under conditions that would allow activation. However, once activated in response to a cross-reacting microbial antigen, these self-reactive lymphocytes can do real damage. In this scenario, the invading microbe substitutes for (mimics) the self antigen for activation. For example, it is believed that rheumatic heart disease, which is a possible complication of a streptococcal throat infection, can result when receptors on helper T cells that recognize streptococcal antigens cross-react with a protein which is present on the tissues that make up the mitral valve of the heart. These cross-reactive Th cells appear to direct an inflammatory response that can severely damage that heart valve.

One reason it has been so difficult to pin down the environmental triggers for most autoimmune diseases is that TCRs which recognize self antigens usually can cross react with multiple environmental antigens. Consequently, although viral or bacterial infections may be involved in some autoimmune disorders, it appears unlikely that any single microbe is responsible for any one autoimmune disease.

Animal models of human autoimmune diseases have been useful for understanding which immune system players are involved, which self antigens are targets of the immune reaction, and which microbial antigens might be involved in the molecular mimicry that may trigger disease. Typically, these models involve animals that have been bred to be exquisitely susceptible to autoimmune disease, or animals whose genes have been altered to make them susceptible. Nevertheless, animal models frequently differ in important respects from the human disease they are meant to model. As a result, many treatments for autoimmune diseases which look promising in an animal model have turned out to be useless in humans.

Inflammation and autoimmune disease

Although molecular mimicry may be responsible for activating lymphocytes that previously had been ignorant of self antigens, there must be more to the story. After all, when self-reactive T cells that have been activated by a microbial mimic reach the tissues, they are in a precarious situation. To avoid apoptotic death by "neglect," they must be continually restimulated, and if they encounter self antigens in an environment that does not provide adequate co-stimulation, they will be anergized or deleted.

As you remember, the innate system usually gives "permission" for the adaptive system to function. Part of this permission involves the activation of antigen presenting cells by inflammatory cytokines such as IFN-γ and TNF which are secreted by cells of the innate system. Once activated, APCs (e.g., macrophages) express the MHC and co-stimulatory molecules required to restimulate T cells which have entered the tissues to do battle. What this means is that when lymphocytes venture out into the tissues to join a war that the innate system is already fighting, restimulation is not a problem. However, for a T cell that recognizes a self antigen which the innate system does not see as dangerous, the tissues can be a very inhospitable place – because a self-reactive lymphocyte usually will not receive the co-stimulation necessary for its survival.

The bottom line is that it is not enough for a microbe to activate self-reactive T cells by mimicry. There also must be an inflammatory reaction going on in the same tissues that express the self antigen. Otherwise it is unlikely that self-reactive lymphocytes would exit the blood into these tissues, and, if they did, that they would survive. This requirement for inflammation at the site of an autoimmune attack helps explains why, for example, a strep infection in the throat only rarely leads to rheumatic heart disease.

So the scenario most immunologists favor for the initiation of autoimmune disease is this: a genetically susceptible individual is attacked by a microbe that activates T cells whose receptors just happen to cross react with a self antigen. Simultaneously, an inflammatory reaction takes place in the tissues where the self antigen is expressed. This inflammation could be caused either by the mimicking microbe itself, or by another, unrelated infection or trauma. As a result of this inflammatory reaction, APCs are activated that can re-stimulate self-reactive T cells. In addition, cytokines generated by the inflammatory response can upregulate class I MHC expression on normal cells in the tissues, making these cells better targets for destruction by self-reactive CTLs.

Examples of autoimmune disease

Autoimmune diseases usually are divided into two groups: organ-specific and multi-system diseases. Let's look at examples of both types, paying special attention to the self antigens against which the autoimmune response is thought to be directed, and to the environmental antigens that may be involved in molecular mimicry.

Insulin-dependent diabetes mellitus is an example of an organ-specific autoimmune disease. In this disease, the targets of autoimmune attack are the insulin-producing "β cells" of the pancreas. Although antibodies produced by self-reactive B cells may participate in the chronic inflammation that contributes to the pathology of this disease, it is currently believed that the initial attack on the β cells is mediated by CTLs.

Clearly, there are genetic factors that help determine susceptibility to diabetes, since the probability that both identical twins will suffer from this autoimmune disease is about 50% if one of them has it. It is known, for example, that some individuals have a version of the gene for CTLA-4 which is associated with an increased risk of type 1 diabetes. Patients with this variant make less CTLA-4 RNA and presumably are less able to limit the activity of self-reactive T cells that recognize β cell antigens.

Thus far, no strong candidates have emerged for environmental factors that might trigger the initial attack on β cells. However, many immunologists believe that diabetes (and, perhaps, other autoimmune diseases) results, at least in part, when natural regulatory T cells (nTregs), which should help keep potentially self-reactive CTLs under control, don't function properly. Unfortunately, it remains to be discovered exactly how these regulatory T cells accomplish this feat.

In diabetes, destruction of insulin-producing cells in the pancreas usually begins months or even years before the first symptoms of diabetes appear, so this disease is sometimes referred to as a "silent killer." Indeed, by the time symptoms appear, more than 90% of a patient's β cells usually will have been destroyed. Fortunately, antibodies that bind to β cell antigens are produced very early in the disease. As a result, relatives of diabetic patients can be tested to determine whether they might be in the early stages of diabetes, and could be helped by early intervention. This is important, because if a child has a sibling who developed diabetes early in life, and if that child's immune system makes antibodies that recognize β cell proteins, the probability that he will develop diabetes within the next five years is nearly 100%.

Myasthenia gravis is an autoimmune disease that results when self-reactive antibodies bind to the receptor for an important neurotransmitter, acetylcholine. When the message that is normally carried by acetylcholine from nerve to muscle is not received (because the antibodies interfere with its reception), muscle weakness and paralysis can result. Immunologists have noticed that a region of one of the poliovirus proteins is similar in amino acid sequence to part of the acetylcholine receptor protein, so it is possible that a polio infection might provide one mimic which could activate lymphocytes whose receptors cross-react with the acetylcholine receptor.

Multiple sclerosis is an inflammatory disease of the central nervous system that is thought to be initiated by self-reactive T cells. In multiple sclerosis, chronic inflammation destroys the myelin sheaths that are required for nerve cells in the brain to transmit electrical signals efficiently, causing defects in sensory inputs (e.g., vision) and paralysis. Macrophages recruited by cytokines secreted by T cells are thought to play a major role in causing this inflammation. At first there was a question as to how T cells could get into the brain to initiate this disease, but eventually it was discovered that activated T cells (but not virgin T cells) can cross the blood–brain barrier. The presumed target of these T cells is a major component of the myelin sheath: myelin basic protein. T cells isolated from multiple sclerosis patients can recognize a peptide derived from myelin basic protein as well as peptides derived from proteins encoded by both herpes simplex virus and Epstein–Barr virus (the virus that causes mononucleosis). So a possible scenario is that when genetically susceptible individuals are infected with herpes virus or Epstein–Barr virus, they produce T cells that recognize proteins from these viruses. Some of these activated T cells may have receptors that cross-react with myelin basic protein, and once these T cells cross the blood–brain barrier, they can lead the attack on the myelin sheaths, causing the symptoms of multiple sclerosis.

Of course, very few people who have Epstein–Barr or herpes infections get multiple sclerosis, so exposure to microbial mimics is not the whole story. Indeed, as is true of most autoimmune diseases, multiple sclerosis has a strong genetic component: it is about ten times more probable that identical twins will share this disease than it is for non-identical twins to both be afflicted. In addition, it is about 20 times more likely that the nonidentical twin of someone with multiple sclerosis also will have the disease than it is for a person in the general population. There also are certain "resistant" groups (e.g., Hispanic, Asian, and Native American) who have relatively low rates of multiple sclerosis, presumably because of their particular genetic makeup. However, the only gene that has been shown conclusively to confer increased susceptibility to multiple sclerosis is a particular class II MHC gene.

Rheumatoid arthritis is a systemic autoimmune disease that is characterized by chronic inflammation of the joints. One of the presumed targets of this autoimmune reaction is a certain cartilage protein, and T cells from arthritic patients can recognize both the cartilage protein and a protein encoded by the bacterium that causes tuberculosis. Moreover, mice injected with *Mycobacterium tuberculosis* suffer from inflammation of the joints, suggesting, but not proving, that a mycobacterial infection may trigger rheumatoid arthritis in some patients.

IgM antibodies that can bind to the Fc region of IgG antibodies are found in the joints of individuals with rheumatoid arthritis. These antibodies can form IgM–IgG antibody complexes, which can activate macrophages that have entered the joints, increasing the inflammatory reaction. Indeed, the inflammation associated with rheumatoid arthritis is caused mainly by tumor necrosis factor produced by macrophages that infiltrate the joints under the direction of self-reactive helper T cells. To treat arthritis, several drugs are currently being used which "soak up" TNF. One type is an antibody that binds to TNF and prevents it from working, while another is a fake receptor for TNF. Both of these "blockade" strategies are very effective in decreasing the severity of the symptoms experienced by patients with rheumatoid arthritis.

Finally, **lupus erythematosus** is a systemic autoimmune disease that affects about 250 000 people in the United States, roughly 90% of whom are women. This disease can have multiple manifestations including a red rash on the forehead and cheeks (giving the "red wolf" appearance for which the disease was named), inflammation of the lungs, arthritis, kidney damage, hair loss, paralysis, and convulsions. Lupus is caused by a breakdown in both B and T cell tolerance that results in the production of a diverse collection of IgG antibodies which recognize a wide range of self antigens, including DNA, DNA–protein complexes, and RNA–protein complexes. These autoantibodies can form self antigen–antibody complexes which "clog" organs in the body that contain "filters" (e.g., kidneys, joints, and the brain), causing chronic inflammation.

Non-identical twins have about a 2% probability of both having lupus if one twin has the disease. With identical twins, this probability increases about ten-fold. This indicates a strong genetic component to the disease, and more than a dozen MHC and non-MHC genes have been identified, each of which seems to slightly increase the probability that a person will contract lupus. Although no specific microbial infection has been associated with the initiation of this autoimmune disease, mice that lack functional genes for Fas or Fas ligand exhibit lupus-like symptoms. This has led immunologists to speculate that lupus may involve a defect in activation-induced cell death, in which lymphocytes that should die due to chronic stimulation survive to cause the disease. There is also some evidence that humans with mutations which increase the sensitivity of their Toll-like receptors to RNA and DNA are lupus-prone.

THOUGHT QUESTIONS

1. Describe the events that lead to the degranulation of mast cells during an allergic reaction.

2. Why do some people have allergies, whereas others do not?

3. What events are likely to be required to initiate an autoimmune reaction?

LECTURE 13
Immunodeficiency

REVIEW

Most of the time, the immune system functions flawlessly. Nevertheless, it occasionally "makes mistakes." Some of these mistakes are the result of special situations in which the system functions as designed, but the response to the invader either is misguided or over exuberant.

Allergies result when the immune system overproduces IgE antibodies in response to environmental antigens (allergens). Immunologists are not sure what causes this misguided response. Their best thought is that a defect in immune regulation causes production of large numbers of allergen-specific Th2 cells. These helper T cells then orchestrate the overproduction of allergen-specific IgE antibodies. Atopic individuals frequently inherit a genetic predisposition to allergies, and the timing and extent of exposure to microbial infections may influence whether susceptible individuals become atopic.

Autoimmunity results when the mechanisms designed to enforce tolerance of self antigens don't function properly.

Again, immunologists don't know exactly why this happens. Clearly, for autoimmunity to occur, a person must have MHC molecules which can present self antigens, and lymphocytes with receptors which can recognize these antigens. So there is a genetic component. In addition, it is believed that environmental factors are involved, but what these factors might be has been difficult to discover – probably because there are many of them. The current best hypothesis is that autoimmunity can be triggered when an invading microbe "mimics" a self antigen. According to this scenario, the microbe activates lymphocytes which have receptors that recognize both a microbial antigen and a self antigen. Once activated in response to the microbial invasion, these cross-reactive lymphocytes mount an attack on both the invader and the cells or proteins of the infected individual.

Serious disease may result when our immune system does not operate at full strength. Some of these immunodeficiencies are caused by genetic defects that disable parts of the immune network. Others are "acquired" as the consequence of malnutrition, deliberate immunosuppression (e.g., during organ transplantation or chemotherapy for cancer), or disease (e.g., AIDS).

GENETIC DEFECTS LEADING TO IMMUNODEFICIENCY

A genetic defect, in which a single gene is mutated, can lead to immune system weakness. For example, individuals who are born with non-functional CD40 or CD40L proteins are unable to mount a T cell-dependent antibody response – because T cells either cannot deliver or B cells cannot receive this all-important, co-stimulatory signal. Both class switching and somatic hypermutation require co-stimulation by CD40L, so one result of the CD40–CD40L defect is that B cells secrete mainly IgM antibodies which have not affinity matured.

Other genetic deficiencies affect the formation of the thymus. In one such deficiency, **DiGeorge syndrome**, essentially all thymic tissue is missing, and people with this disorder are susceptible to life-threatening infections because they lack functional T cells.

How the Immune System Works, Fourth Edition. Lauren Sompayrac. © 2012 John Wiley & Sons, Ltd. Published 2012 by John Wiley & Sons, Ltd.

Genetic defects also can knock out both T and B cells. This group of diseases is called **severe combined immunodeficiency syndrome (SCIDS)** – where the "combined" label indicates that neither T nor B cells function properly. It was this disease that forced David Vetter, the famous "bubble boy," to live for 12 years in a pathogen-free, plastic bubble. Although a number of different mutations can result in SCIDS, the best-studied mutation causes a defect in a protein that initiates the gene splicing required to produce B and T cell receptors. Without their receptors, B and T cells are totally useless.

Immunodeficiencies also can result from genetic defects in the innate immune system. For example, people who are born with mutations in important complement proteins (e.g., C3) have lymph nodes with an abnormal architecture (no germinal centers) and B cells which produce mainly IgM antibodies.

Given the large number of different proteins that are involved in making the innate and adaptive immune systems work effectively, it's pretty amazing that mutations leading to immunodeficiency are so rare. In fact, inherited immunodeficiencies afflict only about one in 10000 newborns. It is likely, however, that many other cases of genetic immunodeficiency go undetected because our functionally redundant immune system has evolved to provide "backups" when elements of the main system are disabled.

AIDS

Although genetic immunodeficiencies are relatively rare, millions of people suffer from immunodeficiencies that are acquired. A large group of immunodeficient humans acquired their deficiency when they were infected with the AIDS virus – a virus that currently infects over 30 million people worldwide, with at least three million new infections occurring each year. The AIDS symptoms that originally alerted physicians that they were dealing with a disease which had immunodeficiency as its basis was the high incidence of infections (e.g., *Pneumocystis carinii* pneumonia) or cancers (e.g., Kaposi sarcoma) that usually were only seen in immunosuppressed individuals. Soon, the virus that caused this immunodeficiency was isolated and named the human immunodeficiency virus number one (HIV-1). Currently, this is the world's most intensely studied virus, with nearly a billion dollars being spent annually to try to discover its secrets.

An HIV-1 infection

The early events in a human HIV-1 infection are not well characterized because the infection typically is not diagnosed until weeks or months after exposure to the virus. However, the emerging picture is that these infections typically begin when the virus penetrates the rectal or vaginal mucosa and infects helper T cells which lie below these protective surfaces. The virus uses these cells' biosynthetic machinery to make many more copies of itself, and the newly made viruses then infect other cells. So in the early stages of infection, the virus multiplies relatively unchecked while the innate system gives it its best shot, and the adaptive system is being mobilized. After a week or so, the adaptive system starts to kick in, and virus-specific B cells, helper T cells, and CTLs are activated, proliferate, and begin to do their thing. Consequently, during this early, "acute" phase of a viral infection, there is a dramatic rise in the number of viruses in the body (the "viral load") as the virus multiplies in infected cells. This is followed by a marked decrease in the viral load as virus-specific CTLs go to work.

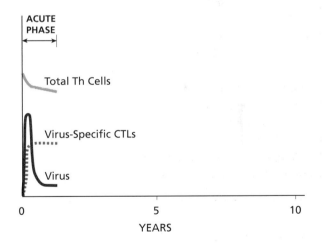

With many viruses (e.g., smallpox), the end result of the acute phase of a viral infection is "sterilization": The immune system destroys all the invading viruses, and memory B and T cells are produced to protect against a subsequent infection by the same virus. In contrast, a full-blown HIV-1 infection always leads to a "chronic" phase that can last for ten or more years. During this phase, a fierce struggle goes on between the immune system and the AIDS virus – a struggle which the virus almost always wins.

During the chronic phase of infection, viral loads decrease to low levels compared with those reached during the height of the acute phase, but the number of virus-specific CTLs and Th cells remains high – a sign that the immune system is still trying hard to defeat the virus.

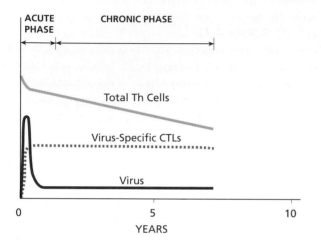

However, as the chronic phase progresses, the total number of Th cells slowly decreases, because these cells are killed as a consequence of the viral infection. Eventually there are not enough Th cells left to provide the help needed by virus-specific CTLs. When this happens, the number of these CTLs also begins to decline, and the viral load increases – because there are too few CTLs left to cope with newly infected cells.

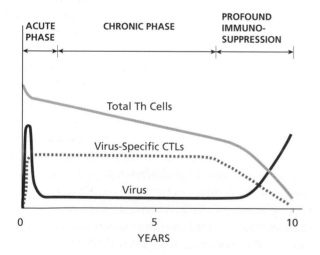

In the end, the immune defenses are overwhelmed, and the resulting profound state of immunosuppression leaves the patient open to unchecked infections by pathogens that normally would not be the slightest problem for a person with an intact immune system. Sadly, these "opportunistic" infections can be lethal to an AIDS patient whose immune system has been destroyed.

HIV-1 versus the immune system

Why is HIV-1 able to defeat an immune system that is so successful in protecting us from most other pathogens? There are two parts to this answer. The first has to do with the nature of the virus itself. All viruses are basically pieces of genetic information (either DNA or RNA) with a protective coat. For the AIDS virus, this genetic information is in the form of RNA which, after the virus enters its target cell, is copied by a viral enzyme (reverse transcriptase) to make a piece of "copy" DNA (cDNA). Next, the DNA of the cell is cut by another enzyme carried by the virus, and the viral cDNA is inserted into the gap in the cellular DNA. Now comes the nasty part. Once the viral DNA has been inserted into a cell's DNA, it can just sit there, and while the virus is in this "latent" state, the infected cell cannot be detected by CTLs. Recent data suggests that it only takes five to ten days for HIV-1 to initiate a latent infection and establish a reservoir of stealth virus in these "sanctuary" cells. Sometime later, in response to signals that are not fully understood, the latent virus can be "reactivated," additional copies of the virus can be produced, and more cells can be infected by these newly minted viruses.

So **the ability to establish a latent infection which cannot be detected by CTLs is one property of HIV-1 that makes this virus such a problem for the immune system.** But it gets worse. The reverse transcriptase enzyme used to copy the HIV-1 RNA is very error-prone: it makes a "mistake" almost every time it copies a piece of viral RNA. This means that most of the new viruses produced by an infected cell are mutated versions of the virus which originally infected that cell. And some of these mutations may enable the newly made viruses to evade the immune system. For example, the virus can mutate so that a viral peptide that formerly was targeted by a CTL can no longer be recognized, or can no longer be presented by the MHC molecule that the CTL was trained to focus on. In fact, it has been shown that it only takes about ten days for these "escape mutants" to arise. When such mutations occur, that CTL will be useless against cells infected with the mutant virus, and new CTLs which recognize another viral peptide will need to be activated. Meanwhile, the virus that has escaped from surveillance by the obsolete CTLs is replicating like crazy, and every time it infects a new cell, it mutates again. Consequently, **the mutation rate of the AIDS virus is so** high that it can usually stay one step ahead of CTLs or antibodies directed against it.

So two of the properties of HIV-1 that make it especially deadly are its ability to establish an undetectable, latent infection, and its high mutation rate. But that's only half the story. The other part has to do with the cells HIV-1 infects. This virus specifically targets cells of the immune system: helper T cells, macrophages, and dendritic cells. The "docking" protein that HIV-1 binds to when it infects a cell is CD4, the co-receptor protein found in large numbers on the surface of helper T cells. This protein also is expressed on macrophages and dendritic cells, although they have fewer CD4 molecules on their surface. By attacking these cells, the AIDS virus either disrupts their function, kills the cells, or makes them targets for killing by CTLs that recognize them as being virus-infected. So the very cells that are needed to activate CTLs and to provide them with help are damaged or destroyed by the virus.

Even more insidiously, HIV-1 can turn the immune system against itself by using processes which are essential for immune function to spread and maintain the viral infection. For example, HIV-1 can attach to the surface of dendritic cells and be transported by these cells from the tissues, where there are relatively few CD4$^+$ cells, into the lymph nodes, where huge numbers of CD4$^+$ T cells are located. Not only are there helper T cells within easy reach in the lymph nodes, many of these cells are proliferating, making them ideal candidates to be infected and become HIV-1 "factories."

Also, AIDS viruses that have been opsonized either by antibodies or by complement are retained in lymph nodes by follicular dendritic cells. This display is intended to help activate B cells. However, CD4$^+$ T cells also pass through these forests of follicular dendritic cells, and as they do, they can be infected by the opsonized AIDS viruses. And because virus particles typically remain bound to follicular dendritic cells for months, lymph nodes actually become reservoirs of HIV-1. Indeed, HIV-1 takes advantage of the normal trafficking of immune system cells through lymph nodes, and turns these secondary lymphoid organs into its own playground.

In summary, the pathological consequences of an HIV-1 infection are the result of the virus' ability to slowly destroy the immune system of the patient, leading to a state of profound immunosuppression which makes the individual an inviting host for life-threatening infections. The virus is able to do this because it can establish a latent, "stealth" infection, because it has a high mutation rate, because it preferentially infects and disables the immune system cells that normally would defend against it, and because it uses the immune system itself to facilitate its spread throughout the body.

Living with AIDS

Untreated, most people infected with HIV-1 die within ten years. Fortunately, for those who can afford it, chemotherapy (Highly Active Anti-Retroviral Treatment) is now available which targets specific aspects of the viral replication cycle, and can lengthen the life of an AIDS patient by many years. However, this chemotherapy is not without side effects. Indeed, for those on HAART, there is an increased risk for cancer, cognitive disorders, as well as kidney, liver, bone, and heart disease.

Interestingly, the immune system of a small fraction of those infected with HIV-1 (less than 1%) is able to control the infection for a relatively long period of time. In fact, some of these "elite controllers" have almost undetectable levels of virus, and have remained symptom-free for more than 15 years. As you might expect, immunologists are very interested in understanding how the immune system of an elite controller deals with a viral infection that is deadly for most other humans. Although the story is far from complete, there are some clues.

One consistent finding is that innate and adaptive defenses of elite controllers seem to fire up more quickly after the initial infection than does the immune system of "ordinary" humans. Several possible reasons for this quick response have been discovered. For example, the pattern recognition receptors of some elite controllers trigger unusually vigorous secretion of IFN-α and IFN-β by cells of the innate immune system. These "warning cytokines" cause infected cells to die by apoptosis, destroying the viruses that are replicating within them. In addition, IFN-α and IFN-β activate genes within infected cells that encode proteins which limit the efficiency of replication of the AIDS virus.

In Lecture 4, I noted that one reason MHC molecules are so polymorphic is to increase the probability that at least some individuals in the population will have MHC molecules that can bind to and present an invader's peptides. This idea is supported by the finding that certain class I MHC molecules are found much more often in elite controllers than in the general population. The thinking here is that because these MHC molecules efficiently present HIV-1 peptides, killer T cells will be activated earlier in an infection when the number of infected cells is still small. In addition, when CTLs from elite controllers are tested in the laboratory, they tend to be more vicious killers than CTLs from patients who cannot control the infection. This seems to be due to the ability of these "super CTLs" to mobilize the killing enzyme, granzyme B, and to deliver it into its target cells. Again, the thinking is that these CTLs kill faster, and can control the infection before it gets out of hand.

Of course, the hope is that if the unique features of the immune systems of elite controllers can be understood in more detail, this information may be helpful in devising new treatments for persons infected with HIV-1. It is important to understand, however, that elite controllers are still infected. Their immune system has not defeated the virus. It has only controlled it for an extended period of time.

THOUGHT QUESTIONS

1. Describe what happens to a patient's immune system during the course of an HIV-1 infection.

2. Discuss the features of an HIV-1 infection that make it so difficult for the immune system to deal with.

LECTURE 14

Cancer and the Immune System

REVIEW

Mutations which are inherited or which arise spontaneously can cause the immune system to function suboptimally. Indeed about 1 in 10 000 newborns suffer from some form of "genetic" immunodeficiency. Other immunodeficiencies arise when the immune system is suppressed by drugs or disease.

Millions of humans are immunodeficient as a result of infection with the AIDS virus. HIV-1 goes at the immune system "head on" by infecting and destroying the immune warriors which might otherwise defend against the attack. The virus uses the immune system to facilitate its spread throughout the body, and it can establish a chronic, undetectable infection in immune system cells. Consequently, a "hidden" reservoir of virus is maintained within the body of an infected individual. In addition, because the virus mutates rapidly, killer T cells, which can recognize and kill infected cells, quickly become "obsolete," allowing the virus to stay one step ahead of the immune defenses.

Untreated, most AIDS patients succumb to infections which the immune system of a healthy individual could easily defeat. Some "elite controllers" are chronically infected with the virus, but remain asymptomatic for long periods of time. Immunologists are eagerly examining the immune system of these "lucky few" to try to determine why they are able to control an infection which is lethal to so many others.

In this lecture, we're going to discuss how the immune system deals with cancer. This is a disease which will touch us all, either directly or indirectly. Because you may not have had a cancer course, I will begin by discussing some general properties of cancer cells. After all, it's important to know the enemy.

CANCER IS A CONTROL SYSTEM PROBLEM

Cancer arises when multiple control systems within a single cell are corrupted. These control systems are of two basic types: systems that promote cell growth (proliferation), and safeguard systems that protect against "irresponsible" cell growth. When controlled properly, cell proliferation is a good thing. After all, an adult human is made up of trillions of cells, so a lot of proliferation must take place between the time we are a single, fertilized egg and the time we are full-grown. However, once a human reaches adulthood, most cell proliferation ceases. For example, when the cells in your kidney have proliferated to make that organ exactly the right size, kidney cells stop proliferating. On the other hand, skin cells and cells that line our body cavities (e.g., our intestines) must proliferate almost continuously to replenish cells that are lost as these surfaces are eroded by normal wear and tear. All this cell proliferation, from cradle to grave, must be carefully controlled to insure that the right amount of proliferation takes place at the right places in the body and at the right times.

Usually, the growth-promoting systems within our cells work just fine. However, occasionally one of these systems may malfunction, and a cell may begin to proliferate inappropriately. When this happens, that cell has taken the first step toward becoming a cancer cell.

Because these growth-promoting systems are made up of proteins, malfunctions usually occur when a gene that specifies one of these proteins is mutated. **A gene, which when mutated, can cause a cell to proliferate inappropriately is called a proto-oncogene. And the mutated version of such a gene is called an oncogene. The important point here is that uncontrolled cell growth can result when a _normal_ cellular gene is mutated.**

To protect against malfunctions in the control systems that promote cell proliferation, Mother Nature has equipped cells with internal safeguard systems. These safeguards also are composed of proteins, and they are of two general types: systems that help prevent mutations, and systems that deal with these mutations once they occur. For example, cells have a number of different repair systems that can fix damaged DNA, helping safeguard against mutations. These DNA repair systems are especially important, because mutations occur continuously in the DNA of all our cells. In fact, it is estimated that on average, each of our cells suffers about 25 000 mutational events every day. Fortunately, repair systems work non-stop, and if the DNA damage is relatively small, it can be repaired immediately as part of the "maintenance" repair program.

Sometimes, however, the maintenance repair systems may miss a mutation, especially when there are many mutations and the repair systems are overwhelmed. When this happens, a second type of safeguard system comes into play – one that monitors unrepaired mutations. If the mutations are not extensive, this safeguard system stops the cell from proliferating to give the repair systems more time to do their thing. However, if the genetic damage is severe, the safeguard system will trigger the cell to commit suicide, eliminating the possibility that it will become a cancer cell. One of the important components of this safeguard system is a protein called p53. **Proteins like p53, which help safeguard against uncontrolled cell growth, are called tumor suppressors, and the genes that encode them are called anti-oncogenes or tumor suppressor genes.**

Mutations in p53 have been detected in the majority of human tumors, and scientists have now created mice with mutant p53 genes. In contrast to normal mice, which rarely get cancer, mice that lack functional p53 proteins usually die of cancer before they are seven months old. So, if you are ever asked to give up one gene, don't pick p53!

The take-home lesson is that every normal cell has both proto-oncogenes and tumor suppressor genes. Where things get dangerous is when proto-oncogenes are mutated, so that the cell proliferates inappropriately, _and_ tumor suppressor genes are mutated so that the cell can't defend itself against proto-oncogenes "gone wrong." Indeed, **cancer results when _multiple_ control systems, both growth-promoting and safeguard, are corrupted within a single cell.** It is estimated that between four and seven such mutations are required to produce most common cancers. This is the reason why cancer is a disease which generally strikes late in life: it usually takes a long time to accumulate the multiple mutations required to inappropriately activate growth-promoting systems and to disable safeguard systems.

Mutations that affect growth-promoting systems and safeguard systems can occur in any order. For example, one type of mutation that is especially insidious is a genetic alteration which disrupts a safeguard system involved in repairing mutated DNA. When this happens, the mutation rate in a cell can soar, making it much more likely that the cell will accrue the multiple mutations required to turn it into a cancer cell. This type of "mutation-accelerating" defect is found in many (perhaps all) cancer cells. Indeed, **one of the hallmarks of a cancer cell is a genetically unstable condition in which cellular genes are constantly mutating.**

CLASSIFICATION OF CANCER CELLS

Cancer cells can be grouped into two general categories: non-blood-cell cancers (usually referred to as "solid tumors") and blood-cell cancers. Solid tumors are further classified according to the cell type from which they arise. Carcinomas, the most common tumors in humans, are cancers of epithelial cells, and include lung, breast, colon, and cervical cancer, among others. These cancers generally kill by metastasizing to vital organs, where they grow and crowd the organ until it no longer can function properly. **Humans also get cancers of the connective and structural tissues, although these "sarcomas" are relatively rare compared to carcinomas.** Perhaps the best known example of a sarcoma is bone cancer (osteosarcoma).

Blood-cell cancers make up the other class of human cancers, and the most frequent of these are leukemias and lymphomas. Blood-cell cancers arise when descendants of blood stem cells, which normally should mature into lymphocytes or myeloid cells (e.g., neutrophils) stop maturing, and just continue proliferating. In a real sense, these blood cells refuse to "grow up" – and that's the problem. In leukemia, the immature cells fill up the bone marrow and prevent other blood cells from maturing. As a result, the patient usually dies from anemia (due to a scarcity of red blood cells) or from infections (due to a deficit of immune system cells). In lymphoma, large "clusters" of immature cells form in lymph nodes and other secondary lymphoid organs – clusters that in some ways resemble solid tumors. Lymphoma patients usually succumb to infections or organ malfunction.

There is another way to classify human cancers: spontaneous and virus-associated. Most human tumors are called spontaneous, because they arise when a single cell accumulates a collection of mutations that causes it to acquire the properties of a cancer cell. These mutations can result from errors made when cellular DNA is copied to be passed down to daughter cells, or from the effects of mutagenic compounds (carcinogens) that are byproducts of normal cellular metabolism or that are present in the air we breathe and the food we eat. Mutations can also be caused by radiation (including UV light) or by errors made in assembling the segments of DNA that make up the B and T cell receptors. As we go through life, these mutations occur "spontaneously," but there are certain factors that can accelerate the rate of mutation: cigarette smoking, a fatty diet, an increased radiation exposure from living at high altitude, working in a plutonium processing plant, and so on.

In addition to mutations in cellular genes that can corrupt growth-promoting and safeguard systems, some viruses produce proteins that can interfere with the proper functioning of these same systems in virus-infected cells. Virus-associated cancers also are "spontaneous" in the sense that mutations are involved. However, virus-associated cancers have, as an additional accelerating factor, a viral infection. For example, essentially all human cervical cancers involve an infection by the human papilloma virus. This sexually transmitted virus infects cells that line the uterine cervix, and expresses in these cells viral proteins that can disable two safeguard systems, including the p53 system. Likewise, hepatitis B virus can establish a chronic infection of liver cells, can inactivate p53, and can act as an accelerating factor for liver cancer. So the net effect of an infection with these special "tumor" viruses is to decrease the total number of cellular genes that must be mutated to turn a normal cell into a cancer cell.

The hallmark of virus-associated cancer is that only a small fraction of infected individuals actually get cancer, yet for those who do, virus or viral genes usually can be recovered from their tumors. For example, less than 1% of the women infected with genital human papilloma virus will ever get cancer of the cervix, yet human papilloma virus genes have been found in over 90% of all cervical carcinomas examined. The reason for this, of course, is that the virus can't cause cancer by itself – it can only accelerate the process that involves the accumulation of cancer-causing mutations. About one fifth of all human cancers have a viral infection as an accelerating factor.

IMMUNE SURVEILLANCE AGAINST CANCER

From this introduction, it should be clear that powerful defenses exist within the cell (e.g., tumor suppressor proteins) to deal harshly with most wannabe cancer cells. Whether or not the immune system also plays a major role in protecting us against the majority of human cancers is not nearly so clear.

In mice which have been engineered so that one or more of the components of their immune system is defective, an increased incidence of lymphoma, leukemia, and virus-associated cancer is well documented. However, the evidence that mice with compromised immune systems experience an increase in solid tumors that do not involve a virus infection is not compelling. In one study, for example, 12 mutant mice that lacked the RAG-2 protein (which is required to assemble B and T cell receptors) were examined. These mice, which are without functional B and T cells, showed no signs of disease while they were alive. However, autopsies revealed that 11 of them had small intestinal tumors, and one had a small lung tumor. Eleven normal mice, housed under similar conditions, had no tumors. These results, although suggestive, beg the question: if B or T cells really are important for protection against solid tumors, why were almost all of these tumors in the intestines and not in the other places that humans commonly get tumors? These mice were raised in "pathogen-free" conditions, so the bacteria in their intestines were different from the bacteria present in the intestines of ordinary mice. Consequently, it is possible that under these conditions, the combination of an unnatural intestinal flora and the RAG-2 mutation predisposed these mice to intestinal tumors. Moreover, because there are significant differences between mouse and human immune systems, it is difficult to know which experiments with mice are relevant to human cancer.

In humans there is also strong evidence that a weakened immune system can increase one's chances of getting blood-cell and virus-associated cancer. However, the published data do not convincingly support the contention that a compromised immune system leads to an increase in the most common of all human tumors: those that are not of blood-cell origin and which are not virus-associated. For example, one oft-quoted study showed that patients who received heart transplants, and who were immunosuppressed to avoid rejection of their transplanted organ, had rates of lung cancer that were 25 times that of the general population. However, individuals who received other types of transplants (e.g., kidneys), and who also were immunosuppressed, did not experience increased rates of lung cancer. Consequently, the increase in lung cancer in the heart transplant patients might simply reflect the fact that many of the patients in this study were cigarette smokers.

So does the immune system provide significant protection against cancer? To try to answer this question, let's examine the roles which various immune system cells might play in cancer surveillance – keeping in mind that different kinds of cancer may be viewed very differently by these cells.

CTLs and spontaneous tumors

The majority of human cancers are spontaneous tumors that are not of blood-cell origin, and it has been proposed that killer T cells might provide surveillance against these cancers. Let's try to evaluate this possibility.

Imagine that a heavy smoker finally accumulates enough mutations in the cells of his lungs to turn one of them into a cancer cell. Remember, it only takes one bad cell to make a cancer. And let's suppose that because of these mutations, this cell expresses proteins that could be recognized as foreign by CTLs. Now let me ask you a question: where are this man's naive T cells while the tumor is growing in his lung? That's right. They are circulating through the blood, lymph, and secondary lymphoid organs. Do they leave this circulation pattern to enter the tissues of the lung? No, not until after they have been activated.

So right away, in terms of immune surveillance, we have a "traffic problem." To make self tolerance work, Mother Nature set up the traffic system so that naive T cells don't get out into the tissues where they might encounter self antigens that were not present in the thymus during tolerance induction. As a result, it's unlikely that virgin T cells ever would "see" tumor antigens expressed in the lung – because they just don't go there. What we have here is a serious conflict between the need to preserve tolerance of self (and avoid autoimmune disease) and the need to provide surveillance against tumors that arise, as most tumors do, out in the tissues. And tolerance wins.

Now, sometimes virgin T cells do disobey the traffic laws and wander out into the tissues. So you might imagine that this kind of adventure could give some T cells a chance to look at the tumor that's growing in this guy's lung, and be activated. But wait! What is required for T cell activation? First of all, killer T cells must recognize antigens which are produced within a cell and presented by class I MHC molecules on the surface of that cell. This means that the tumor cell itself must do the antigen presentation. So far, so good. However, CTLs also require co-stimulation from the cell that presents the antigen. Is this lung tumor cell going to provide that co-stimulation? I don't think so! This isn't an antigen presenting cell, after all. It's a plain old lung cell, and lung cells usually don't express co-stimulatory molecules like B7. Consequently, if a renegade, virgin CTL breaks the traffic laws, enters the lung, and recognizes a tumor antigen displayed by the tumor cell, that CTL most likely will be anergized or killed – because the tumor cell cannot provide the co-stimulation the CTL needs for survival.

Again we see a conflict between tolerance induction and tumor surveillance. The two-key system of specific recognition plus co-stimulation was set up so that T cells which recognize self antigens out in the tissues, but which do not receive proper co-stimulation, will be anergized or killed to prevent autoimmunity. Unfortunately, this same two-key system makes it very difficult for CTLs to be activated by tumor cells that arise in the tissues. So the bottom line is that a CTL would have to perform "unnatural acts" to be activated by a tumor out in the tissues: it would have to break the traffic laws, and somehow avoid being anergized or killed. This could happen, of course, but it would be very inefficient compared to the activation of CTLs in response to, for example, a viral infection.

Another possible scenario is that cancer cells from the primary tumor might metastasize to a lymph node, where T cells could be activated. However, by the time this happens, the original tumor probably will have become quite large. Even a tumor that weighs only about half an ounce will contain more than 10 billion cancer cells – more cells than there are people on our planet! This poses a major problem for immune surveillance, because cancer cells usually mutate like crazy, and with so many cells mutating, it is likely that some of these mutations will prevent recognition or presentation of tumor antigens. For example, the gene encoding the tumor antigen itself can mutate so that the tumor antigen no longer can be recognized by activated CTLs, or no longer will fit properly into the groove of an MHC molecule for presentation. In addition, tumor cells can mutate so that they stop producing the particular MHC molecules that CTLs are restricted to recognize. This happens quite frequently: about 15% of the tumors that have been examined have lost expression of at least one of their MHC molecules. Also, genes that encode the TAP transporters can mutate in a tumor cell, with the result that tumor antigens will not be efficiently transported for loading onto class I MHC molecules. Indeed, **a tumor cell's high mutation rate is its greatest advantage over the immune system, and usually keeps these cells one step ahead of surveillance by CTLs. So even when it occurs, CTL surveillance is usually a case of "too little, too late."**

CTLs and cancerous blood cells

Okay, so CTLs probably don't provide serious surveillance against non-blood-cell, spontaneous tumors. That's a real bummer, because these make up the majority of human tumors. But what about blood-cell cancers like leukemia and lymphoma? Maybe CTLs are useful against them. After all, immunosuppressed humans do have higher frequencies of leukemia and lymphoma than do humans with healthy immune systems. This suggests that there might be something fundamentally different about the way the immune system views tumors in tissues and organs versus the way it sees blood cells that have become cancerous. Let's take a look at what these differences might be.

One of the problems that CTLs have in providing surveillance against tumors that arise in tissues is that these tumors simply are not on the normal traffic pattern of virgin T cells – and it's hard to imagine how a CTL could be activated by a cancer it doesn't see. In contrast, most blood-cell cancers are found in the blood, lymph, and secondary lymphoid organs, and this is ideal for viewing by CTLs, which pass through these areas all the time. Thus, **in the case of blood-cell cancers, the traffic patterns of cancer cells and virgin T cells actually intersect. Moreover, in contrast to tumors in tissues, which usually are unable to supply the co-stimulation required for activation of virgin T cells, some cancerous blood cells actually express high levels of B7, and therefore can provide the necessary co-stimulation. These properties**

of blood-cell cancers suggest that CTLs may provide surveillance against some of them. Unfortunately, this surveillance must be incomplete, because people with otherwise healthy immune systems still get leukemias and lymphomas.

CTLs and virus-associated tumors

Certain viral infections can predispose a person to particular types of cancer. Because Mother Nature probably designed killer T cells to defend against viral infections, it is easy to imagine that CTLs might provide surveillance against virus-associated tumors. Unfortunately, this surveillance is probably quite limited. Here's why.

Most viruses cause "acute" infections in which all the virus-infected cells are rather quickly destroyed by the immune system. And because a dead cell isn't going to make a tumor, **viruses which only cause acute infections do not play a role in cancer.** This explains why most viral infections are <u>not</u> associated with human cancer.

There are viruses, however, which can evade the immune system, and establish long-term (sometimes lifelong) infections. Importantly, **all viruses which have been shown to play a role in causing cancer are able to establish long-lasting infections during which they "hide" from the immune system.** Because CTLs cannot destroy virus-infected cells while they are hiding, and because these hidden cells are the very ones which eventually become cancer cells, it can be argued that CTLs do not provide effective surveillance against virus-associated cancer.

Of course, you might propose that without killer T cells, more cells would be infected during a virus attack, thereby increasing the number of cells in which the virus might be able to establish a long-term, hidden infection. And this probably is true. In fact, this may help explain why humans with deficient immune systems have higher than normal rates of virus-associated tumors. However, the bottom line is that **CTLs cannot provide significant surveillance against virus-infected cells once they have become cancerous, because these cancers only result from long-term viral infections – infections which CTLs cannot detect or cannot deal with effectively.**

Immune surveillance by macrophages and NK cells

Macrophages and natural killer cells may provide surveillance against some cancers. Hyperactivated macrophages secrete TNF, and express it on their surface. Either form of TNF can kill certain types of tumor cells in the test tube. This brings up an important point: what happens in the test tube is not always the same as what happens in an animal. For example, there are mouse sarcoma cells that are very resistant to killing by TNF in the test tube. In contrast, when mice that have these same sarcomas are treated with TNF, the tumors are rapidly destroyed. Studies of this phenomenon showed that the reason TNF is able to kill the tumor when it is in the animal is that this cytokine actually attacks the blood vessels that feed the tumor, cutting off the blood supply, and causing the tumor cells to starve to death. This type of death is called necrosis, and it was this observation that led scientists to name this cytokine "tumor necrosis factor."

In humans, there are examples of cancer therapies in which activated macrophages are likely to play a major role in tumor rejection. One such therapy involves injecting the tumor with bacille Calmette–Guerin (BCG), a cousin of the bacterium that causes tuberculosis. BCG hyperactivates macrophages, and when it is injected directly into a tumor (e.g., a melanoma), the tumor fills up with highly activated macrophages that can destroy the cancer. In fact, one way of treating bladder cancer is to inject it with BCG – a treatment which is quite effective in eliminating superficial tumors, probably through the action of hyperactivated macrophages.

But how do macrophages tell the difference between normal cells and cancer cells? The answer to this question is not known for certain, but evidence suggests that macrophages recognize tumor cells that have unusual cell surface molecules. One of the duties of macrophages in the spleen is to test red blood cells to see if they have become damaged or old. Macrophages use their sense of "feel" to determine which red cells are past their prime. And when they find an old one, they eat it. What macrophages feel for is a fat molecule called phosphatidylserine. This particular fat is usually found on the inside of young red blood cells, but flips to the outside when the cells get old. Like old red blood cells, tumor cells also tend to have unusual surface molecules, and in fact, some express phosphatidylserine on their surface. It is believed that **the abnormal expression of surface molecules on tumor cells may allow activated macrophages to differentiate between cancer cells and normal cells.**

In the test tube, natural killer cells can destroy some tumor cells. In addition, there is evidence that NK cells can kill cancer cells in the body. **Natural killer cells target cells that express low levels of class I MHC molecules, and which display unusual surface molecules (e.g., proteins which indicate that the target cells are "stressed").**

There would be a number of advantages to having macrophages and NK cells provide surveillance against wannabe cancer cells. First, **unlike CTLs, which take a week or more to get cranked up, macrophages and NK cells are quick-acting.** This is an important consideration, because the longer abnormal cells have to proliferate, the greater is the likelihood they will mutate to take on the characteristics of metastatic cancer cells. In addition, once a tumor becomes large, it is much more difficult for the immune system to deal with. So you would like the weapons that protect against wannabe cancer cells to be ready to go just as soon as the cells start to get a little weird.

You would also like anti-tumor weapons to be focused on diverse targets, because a single target (e.g., the MHC–peptide combination seen by a killer T cell) can be mutated, rendering the target unrecognizable. **Both NK cells and macrophages recognize diverse target structures, so the chances of them being fooled by a single mutation is small. In addition, macrophages are located out in the tissues where most tumors arise, so they can intercept cancer cells at an early stage.** And with immune surveillance, as with real estate, location is everything.

There are problems, however, with macrophages and NK cells providing surveillance against cancer. Macrophages need to be hyperactivated before they can kill cancer cells. That's what the BCG treatments do: they hyperactivate macrophages. So if a wannabe cancer cell arises at a site of inflammation where macrophages are already hyperactivated, that's great. But if there's no inflammatory reaction going on, macrophages will probably remain in a resting state and simply ignore cancer cells. Unlike macrophages, which are found in large numbers in our tissues, most NK cells are found in the blood. Like neutrophils, NK cells are "on call." And the cells which do the calling are activated macrophages and dendritic cells that are responding to an invasion. So again, unless there is an inflammatory reaction going on in the tissues, most NK cells will just continue to circulate in the blood.

As a tumor grows, it eventually becomes so large that the neighboring blood vessels cannot provide the nutrients and oxygen required for continued growth, and some of the cancer cells begin to die. Cancer cells also die when they accumulate mutations that are lethal. Consequently, at a later stage in the growth of a tumor, dying cancer cells may provide the signals required to activate macrophages, which can then recruit natural killer cells from the blood. So at this point, macrophages and NK cells may play a role in destroying at least some of the tumor cells. In addition, because **NK cells do not need to be activated to kill**, natural killer cells that are circulating in the blood may be able to destroy either blood cell cancers or cancer cells that are metastasizing through the blood from a primary tumor.

In summary, **in some circumstances, macrophages and NK cells may provide surveillance against certain types of cancer cells, and the immune system probably is involved in defending against some virus-associated and blood-cell cancers. In addition, the immune system may reduce the frequency of metastases or may help slow the metastatic process once a primary tumor has formed. However, I believe it is unlikely that the immune system provides significant surveillance against most solid tumors in humans during the initial stages of their development. This is my view, but not everyone agrees with me on this point.**

VACCINATION TO PREVENT VIRUS-ASSOCIATED CANCER

One approach which has been successful in using the immune system to prevent cancer is vaccination against tumor viruses. A chronic infection with hepatitis B virus increases one's risk of getting liver cancer about 200-fold, and roughly 20% of long-term, hepatitis B carriers eventually develop this disease. Moreover, hepatitis B virus ranks as one of the most infectious of all viruses: transfer of a fraction of a drop of blood is sufficient to spread the virus from one human to another. Fortunately, vaccines that protect against infection by hepatitis B virus have been available in the United States since 1982, and the current vaccine is administered not only to healthcare professionals, who routinely come into contact with blood and blood products, but also to children. This subunit vaccine gives the immune system a "preview" of a real hepatitis B infection, allowing ample time for memory B cells and the antibodies they produce to be mobilized. Then, if infection does occur, the prepared immune system can quickly eradicate the virus, effectively preventing hepatitis B-associated liver cancer.

Infection with certain "oncogenic" types of human papilloma virus (HPV) can increase the risk of cervical cancer. These viruses are spread by sexual contact, and there are now so many women infected with this virus that cervical carcinoma has become the second most common cancer in women worldwide, resulting in about 250 000 deaths per year.

Although there are about a dozen, slightly different types of HPV that are associated with cervical cancer, two types, HPV-16 and HPV-18, are implicated in about 70% of all cervical cancer cases. Recently, two pharmaceutical companies, Merck and GSK, have pioneered vaccines that are effective in preventing infection by both types of HPV. These are subunit vaccines made from viral coat proteins. In addition, the Merck vaccine includes coat proteins from two other HPV types, HPV-6 and HPV-11, which are not associated with cervical cancer, but which do cause genital warts in both men and women. Their thinking in including these two "extras" is that preventing genital warts might encourage boys and men to be vaccinated, since they might otherwise be reluctant to be vaccinated to prevent a disease (cervical cancer) they cannot get.

Although the Merck and GSK vaccines will be very helpful in decreasing the number of deaths from cervical cancer, a vaccine that would protect against the five HPV types that are most commonly associated with cervical carcinoma could prevent hundreds of thousands of deaths from cancer each year worldwide – providing that most sexually active young women could be vaccinated. Unfortunately, many of the cases of cervical cancer occur in underdeveloped parts of the world, where immunization via injection is problematic.

Although vaccination against infection by cancer-associated viruses is the current star in the effort to enlist the immune system in the battle against cancer, many new approaches are in various stages of testing. We all can hope that these experiments will be successful – because, as it stands now, about one out of every three of us will get cancer during our lifetime.

THOUGHT QUESTIONS

1. There is a conflict between immune surveillance against cancer and the preservation of tolerance of self antigens. Explain.

2. Discuss why the adaptive immune system may provide some surveillance against blood-cell cancers, but not against spontaneous, non-blood-cell cancers.

LECTURE 15

A Critique of the Immune System

REVIEW

Although it is certain that human cells have a number of built-in safeguards to protect them from becoming cancerous, it is not nearly so clear what role the immune system plays in protecting us against this terrible disease – especially in the case of cancers that are not of blood-cell origin, and which do not involve a viral infection. One weapon we might expect would be useful against cancer cells is the killer T cell. After all, these cells are "trained" to look inside other cells to see if there is something wrong in there. However, there are two main problems with CTL surveillance against cancer. The first is that Mother Nature has been very careful to minimize the chances of the immune system attacking our own normal cells, and this requirement conflicts with the possibility of killer T cells destroying cells that "lose it" and become cancerous. T cells are activated in the secondary lymphoid organs, and only after they are activated are they allowed to venture out into the tissues where most tumors are located. Consequently, the normal traffic pattern of naive T cells keeps them from coming into contact with these cancer cells. In addition, most cancer cells cannot supply the co-stimulation required to activate killer T cells, so even a "chance encounter" between a naive T cell and a tumor cell isn't likely to result in activation. Blood cells which become cancerous are more likely to come into contact with naive T cells, but most cancerous blood cells also can't provide the co-stimulation required for T cell activation.

A second problem with killer T cells providing surveillance against cancer is that cancer cells usually have a very high mutation rate. Consequently, even if CTLs are activated in response to a particular cancer cell, it is very likely that there are other cells within the tumor which have mutated so that they are now invisible to those CTLs. As a result, although killer T cells may destroy some cells within a tumor, there usually are other cells there which they cannot kill.

Natural killer cells and macrophages can recognize and kill some tumor cells – those which have unusual molecules on their surface – so these two weapons may be useful against certain types of cancer. NK cells and macrophages have the advantage that they do not take weeks to be activated and to build up their numbers, as CTLs do. However, although macrophages are stationed out in the tissues where most cancers arise, and therefore are in the right place to provide surveillance, resting macrophages are oblivious to cancer cells. In order for a macrophage to become a cancer killer, it must be activated – something that usually happens in response to an infection, not to a cancer cell. Normally, there are very few natural killer cells out in the tissues. Like neutrophils, they are "on call" from the blood, and the innate system cells that usually do the calling are activated macrophages and dendritic cells. Consequently, even though NK cells and macrophages might be capable of destroying cancer cells, these weapons generally are not mobilized efficiently when a cancer begins to form. Later, when the tumor has grown, and cancer cells begin to die due to mutations or the lack of a sufficient blood supply, macrophages may be alerted and NK cells may be recruited from the blood. But by then, it is usually too late.

WE ARE UNDER ATTACK!

Imagine for a moment that the United States is under attack. Large numbers of troops are assembled on our northern and southern borders, armed with a complete array of weaponry from small arms to tanks to warplanes – and they are staging relentless attacks by ground and air. In the Pacific, the Atlantic, and the Gulf of Mexico, warships of every description are on station with guns and missiles trained on our mainland, and enemy airplanes and helicopters are flying unending sorties against our cities. What sort of defense system could possibly protect us against such a never-ending siege, while allowing us to continue doing "business as usual," giving little or no thought to the dangers surrounding us? To provide this level of protection, a defense system would have to do the following:

Protect a large perimeter. Because an attack might come from any direction, our defense system would need to provide protection everywhere along the roughly 9000 mile perimeter of the continental United States.

Defend against simultaneous attacks. Clever foes will attack simultaneously at many different locations, so we must be able to mount a multi-front defense.

Maintain good communication between our forces. In a multi-front war, establishing efficient lines of communication would be key.

Detect individual attacks along the perimeter as soon as they are initiated, and determine the size and composition of the assault force, as well as the location of the invasion. Complete intelligence on the enemy would need to be gathered continually all along the perimeter, and conveyed quickly to command centers from which the proper weapons could be deployed.

Dispatch appropriate weapons to the location where an invasion is taking place. Because we would be defending our country on many fronts, insuring that the right weapons reach the right places would be a significant logistical challenge.

Provide sufficient firepower around the perimeter to delay the advance of attackers until more powerful weapon systems can be mobilized. It would take a while to deploy weapons to specific battle sites, so forces along the perimeter would need to buy time until reinforcements could be sent.

Defend against a variety of different weapons. Our adversary will employ many different weapons systems (e.g., tanks or submarine-based missiles). Consequently, we would need to be ready to deal with whatever they might throw at us.

Respond quickly to invaders armed with "ordinary" weapons. We should already have weapons in our arsenal that can defend against the weapons we know the enemy will be using.

React to invaders armed with novel weapons by quickly producing new counter-weapons. The enemy will be evolving new weapon systems that our defenders have not encountered before. Consequently, we must be "adaptable," having the ability to respond to novel weapons by producing and deploying new defenses.

Mount a proportionate response. If the enemy is attacking us with machine guns, we would not want to respond with nuclear weapons.

Have redundant defense systems. Clever foes will devise ways to disable some of our defense systems (e.g., by jamming one particular radio frequency), so we would need backups.

Insure a high level of cooperation between our various defenses. If our defenders (e.g., the Navy Seals and the Air Force) cooperate, they would be much more effective than if they worked independently.

Learn from experience and fine-tune our defenses. Not only should our armed forces "remember" which weapon systems were effective against a given invader, they must be able to "upgrade" these weapons to better respond to a similar attack at a later time.

Protect our own people against injury by friendly fire. Mounting a powerful defense without causing collateral damage either to our own troops or to our civilians would be a difficult challenge.

Recall or inactivate weapons when each battle is over. Once the enemy has been repulsed at one location, maintaining large stores of weapons at that site would not be economical.

CRITIQUING THE IMMUNE DEFENSE

As I'm sure you understand, the requirements for defending against this hypothetical attack on our country are very similar to the demands made on our immune system as it protects us against the foes we face every day. So as a way of reviewing, let's evaluate how well the human immune system meets these requirements.

Our immune system must defend a large perimeter against simultaneous attacks on multiple fronts. To accomplish this, innate system cells (e.g., macrophages) are stationed beneath every surface that is exposed to the outside world, so we have defenders ready to repulse an attack, wherever it may occur. If the invasion is more serious than those sentinel cells can take care of by themselves, large numbers of reinforcements (e.g., neutrophils and natural killer cells) can be recruited very quickly from nearby blood vessels to help with the defense.

As the battle rages, dendritic cells collect information on the type, size, and location of the attack, and convey this intelligence to nearby secondary lymphoid organs, which function as command centers. There, circulating B cells and T cells can be mobilized. Importantly, these responses are local: only those cells which are present in the neighborhood of the invasion will be affected, and only a limited number of secondary lymphoid organs (e.g., nearby lymph nodes) will be involved. Consequently, many different battles can be fought simultaneously against diverse attackers at various sites around the body.

The number of immune system weapons which are pressed into service will depend on the size of the attack, so the immune system mounts a response which is proportional to the threat. Once activated, most of the weapons of the immune system have a short lifetime, so that once the enemy has been vanquished, obsolete weapons are not left behind on the battlefield to cause trouble. In addition, there are mechanisms in place which deactivate weapons like killer T cells, which are not inherently short-lived. Together, these features insure that when the battle has been won, most of the troops will "stand down," and the former battleground will return to normal.

There is excellent communication between the various arms of the immune defense. Warriors of the innate and adaptive systems communicate by exchanging cytokines, and the immune defense is spatially organized by adhesion molecules and chemokines, which tell the various defenders where to go. These features insure that the appropriate weapons are mobilized and sent to the correct places.

Our immune system has a variety of weapons it can deploy, depending on the enemy. In its arsenal are "conventional" weapons which are designed to defend against invaders we can expect to encounter in the course of a normal lifetime. This weaponry includes cells like macrophages, neutrophils, and natural killer cells, as well as the complement system of proteins.

B cells and T cells have receptors which are assembled using a mix-and-match strategy, and are so diverse that they can recognize and deal with essentially any invader.

Consequently, the adaptive immune system is able to defend against invaders we have never encountered before – or novel weapons which an enemy may be deploying for the first time. Killer T cells specialize in destroying infected cells, and B cells make antibodies that tag invaders for destruction by immune system cells and the complement system. Also, some antibodies can bind to invaders in such a way as to prevent them from infecting cells.

There is a high level of cooperation between the "troops" of the innate and adaptive systems, resulting in a combined defense which is much more potent than would be possible if the two systems, or individual components of the innate and adaptive systems, acted independently. In addition, the immune system is highly redundant, with more than one weapon being useful against a given invader. Consequently, if an attacker mounts a successful defense against one aspect of the immune system, other weapons usually are available to deal with the attack.

The immune system also learns from experience. Over the millennia during which humans have been exposed to various pathogens, the innate system has evolved pattern recognition receptors which remember what these attackers look like. This memory is hard-wired. In contrast to the innate system, which remembers old invaders, the memory of the adaptive system is updatable, so that it can remember recent invaders – those we have encountered during our own lifetime. After an initial attack, memory B and T cells remain, increasing the number of weapons that can be mobilized quickly in the case of a subsequent attack. Moreover, memory B cells usually have receptors that have been fine-tuned to allow them to detect a subsequent invasion by the same foe at an earlier stage – when there are fewer attackers to deal with. In addition, B cells can switch the class of antibodies they produce to insure that they are ready with exactly the right armaments if the invader attacks again. By learning from experience, the adaptive immune system is ready to respond with increased speed and potency to a subsequent attack.

The immune system also goes to great lengths to protect us from friendly fire. The conventional weapons of the innate immune system have evolved over millions of years to focus either on signatures of invaders which have no human counterparts, or on surfaces which are not protected from attack – as are the surfaces of human cells. B cells and T cells undergo rigorous screening to eliminate those with receptors that can recognize our own self molecules. Moreover, B and T cells are mobilized on demand, employing a fail-safe strategy which insures that rogue B or T cells don't decide unilaterally to attack our own molecules. The result of all these precautions is that although the immune system can protect us against almost any threat, serious autoimmune disease is relatively rare.

Finally, because the immune system reacts so quickly, both to common invaders and to uncommon foes we have encountered previously, we usually don't even realize we are under attack. This allows us to do "business as usual" with little regard to the many enemies which seek to do us harm.

WEAKNESSES OF THE IMMUNE SYSTEM

Although the immune system does a wonderful job of protecting us against continual, multi-front attacks by invaders brandishing many kinds of weapons, our defense system does have some weaknesses.

The adaptive immune system reacts relatively slowly to attacks, because its weapons must be produced on demand. Consequently, a novel invader, which is not included in the innate system's catalogue of dangers, sometimes can get a foothold in the body before the adaptive immune system can be mobilized. Such invaders can establish chronic, in some cases lifelong, infections.

Also, there is a conflict between the requirement that our immune system be tolerant of our own self molecules and the need for this system to destroy cancer cells. Indeed, by designing a system that puts a premium on avoiding autoimmune disease, Mother Nature compromised the immune system's ability to defend against cancer. In some cases, there may also be a conflict between protection against autoimmunity and the defense against certain infectious diseases. For example, a mutation in one of the Fc receptor proteins predisposes humans to the autoimmune disease, lupus erythematosus. This mutation is found quite frequently in African populations, and has been shown to protect against the severe effects of malaria – a major cause of childhood death in Africa.

Allergies plague many humans, and this ailment mainly results from the misapplication of an immune system that was designed to defend against parasitic infections. Indeed, it would appear that the potential for allergic reactions is the price we must pay for having weapons such as mast cells and IgE antibodies which can defend us against parasites.

Finally, our immune system functions less well as we age. For example, B cells are produced more or less continuously throughout the lifetime of a human, but the production of virgin T cells decreases as a person ages. The reason for this is that the organ in which T cells mature, the thymus, steadily decreases in activity after puberty, so fewer and fewer freshly minted T cells roll off the thymic assembly line as we get older. That's one reason why some viral diseases, such as mumps, which are just a nuisance to a kid, can be deadly serious to an older person.

BAD DESIGN?

One might argue that the immune system should have been "designed" so that B and T cells could be activated more quickly. After all, there are so few naive B or T cells with receptors which can recognize a given invader that these cells must proliferate for a week or two before there are enough of them to mount a serious defense. This could have been "fixed" by making B and T cell receptors less diverse – so that there would be more naive cells with each particular kind of receptor. However, decreasing the diversity of B and T cell receptors could leave a "hole in our coverage," so that there might not be B or T cells with receptors which could recognize some deadly new pathogen. I don't know this for sure, but I suspect that during evolution, the number of possible different B and T cell receptors was "adjusted" to provide complete coverage without being overly diverse. Probably those early humans whose receptors were not diverse enough were killed by some new pathogen. And those whose receptors were more diverse than are required for a complete defense likely died because their primitive adaptive systems took too long to crank up. My guess is that our fully evolved adaptive immune system has a "Goldilocks" receptor diversity – "just right" to provide maximum protection.

Now, before we accuse Mother Nature of bad design, we also should remember that the immune system did not evolve to protect people living in a modern society. It evolved to protect cavemen. For example, it is unlikely that allergies were an issue for early humans. Those folks were not blessed with the good hygiene we have today, and cavechildren were exposed at an early age to infectious diseases that most likely "deviated" their reaction to allergens away from the abnormal production of IgE antibodies. In fact, while many of us "modern humans" curse IgE antibodies, cavemen would have depended heavily on IgE antibodies to defend against the many parasites which must have plagued them. Indeed, even today, parasitic worms infect roughly a third of the human population.

Cancer also was not a major worry for cavemen. They simply didn't live long enough to have a high probability of contracting this disease. So for them, a system that sacrificed a robust defense against cancer in favor of protection against autoimmune disease (which can be devastating to a young person) made perfect sense. Likewise, it would not have mattered to cavemen that the potency of the immune system declines slowly with age. There were very few elderly cavemen – or cavewomen.

Earlier I mentioned a possible conflict between the defense against some infections (e.g., malaria) and protection against autoimmune disease (e.g., lupus). It is interesting to note that although Americans of African descent who have the Fc receptor mutation which is protective against malaria do have a higher risk of contracting lupus, people with this mutation who actually reside in Africa do not have an increased incidence of lupus! This again illustrates the point that living in an environment (e.g., modern society) which is different from the environment in which our immune system evolved to protect us can give the immune defense a "bad name."

So is it bad design? I don't think so. In fact, although it has a few weaknesses, our immune system is amazingly effective at protecting us against almost any pathogen. Good job, Mother Nature!

Glossary

ADCC: Antibody-dependent cellular cytotoxicity. Antibodies bind to the target, and Fc receptors on the surfaces of cytotoxic cells (e.g., macrophages or NK cells) bind to the Fc portion of the antibodies to form a "bridge" between the target and the cytotoxic cell: antibody-directed killing by cells of the innate system.

Allergen: An antigen that causes allergies.

Anergy: A state of non-functionality.

Anergize: To "neuter" – to render non-functional.

Antigen: A rather loosely used term for the target (e.g., a viral protein) of an antibody or a T cell. To be more precise, an antibody binds to a <u>region</u> of an antigen called the epitope, and the T cell receptor binds to a peptide that is a <u>fragment</u> of an antigen.

Anti-oncogene: A gene that encodes a tumor suppressor protein.

Autophagy: A process by which cells that are starved for nutrients can recycle cytoplasmic components.

APC: Antigen presenting cell. A cell (e.g., an activated macrophage, an activated dendritic cell, or an activated B cell) that can present antigen efficiently to T cells via MHC molecules, and which can supply the co-stimulatory molecules required to activate T cells.

Apoptosis: The process during which cells commit suicide in response to problems within the cell or to signals from outside the cell.

BCR: B cell receptor.

β2-microglobulin: The non-polymorphic chain of the class I MHC molecule.

Central memory cells: Memory B or T cells that reside in the secondary lymphoid organs and proliferate slowly. The progeny of these cells resupply long-lived plasma B cells and memory effector T cells which have died of old age. If there is a second attack, central memory cells quickly produce short-lived plasma B cells (which secrete antibodies) and effector T cells (which travel to the tissues to participate in the battle).

Central tolerance induction: Process by which T cells with receptors that recognize abundant self antigens in the thymus are anergized or deleted.

Chemokine: A special cytokine that is used to direct cells to their proper positions.

Clonal selection principle: When receptors on B or T cells recognize their cognate antigen, these cells are triggered (selected) to proliferate. As a result, a clone of B or T cells with identical antigen specificities is produced.

Cognate antigen: The antigen (e.g., a bacterial protein) which a B or T cell's receptors recognize and bind to.

Co-receptor: The CD4 or CD8 molecules on T cells, or the complement receptor on B cells. Ligation of the co-receptors amplifies the signal sent through the B or T cell receptors.

Cortical thymic epithelial cell: Cells in the cortex of the thymus which are the "examiners" during positive selection (MHC restriction) of T cells which recognize MHC–peptide complexes.

Co-stimulation: The second "key" that B and T cells need for activation.

Crosslink: Cluster together (e.g., an antigen may crosslink a B cell's receptors).

Cross-presentation: A process by which exogenous proteins, which normally should be presented by class II MHC molecules, are presented by class I MHC molecules.

Cross-reacts: Recognizes several different epitopes. For example, a B cell's receptors may bind to (cross-react with) several different epitopes that are present on several different antigens.

CTL: Cytotoxic lymphocyte. Synonym for killer T cell.

Cytokines: Hormone-like messenger molecules that cells use to communicate.

Cytokine profile: The mixture of different cytokines that a cell secretes.

Cytoplasm: The liquid portion of a cell in which the organelles and the nucleus "float."

Dendritic cell (DC): A starfish-shaped cell which, when activated by battle signals, travels from the tissues to the secondary lymphoid organs to present antigen to naive T cells.

DTH: Delayed type hypersensitivity. An inflammatory reaction in which Th cells recognize a specific invader, and secrete cytokines that activate and recruit innate system cells to do the killing.

Elite controller: A person infected with HIV-1 whose immune system is able to control the infection for an extended period of time.

Endocytosis: Similar to phagocytosis except that it begins when the thing being "eaten" binds to a receptor on the surface of the phagocytic cell: receptor-initiated phagocytosis.

Endogenous protein: A protein that is produced within the cell in question – the opposite of an exogenous protein.

Endoplasmic reticulum: A large sack-like structure inside the cell from which most proteins destined for transport to the cell surface begin their journey.

Endothelial cells: Cells shaped like shingles that line the insides of our blood vessels.

Epithelial cells: Cells that form part of the barrier that separates our bodies from the outside world.

Epitope: The region of an antigen that is recognized by a B or T cell's receptors.

Exogenous protein: A protein that is found outside the cell in question – the opposite of an endogenous protein.

Follicular dendritic cell (FDC): A starfish-shaped cell that retains opsonized antigens in germinal centers, and displays these antigens for B cells.

Germinal center: An area in a secondary lymphoid organ in which B cells proliferate, undergo somatic hypermutation, and switch classes. Also known as a "secondary lymphoid follicle."

Hc: Heavy chain protein of the antibody molecule.

High endothelial venule (HEV): A region in a blood vessel where there are high endothelial cells which allow lymphocytes to exit the blood.

IFN-γ: Interferon gamma. A cytokine secreted mainly by Th1 helper T cells and NK cells.

Inducible regulatory T cells (iTregs): CD4$^+$ T cells which produce cytokines that can negatively regulate the immune response out in the tissues.

Inflammatory response: A rather general term that describes the battle that macrophages, neutrophils, and other immune system cells wage against an invader.

Interleukin: A protein (cytokine) that is used for communication between leukocytes (e.g., IL-2).

Isotype: A synonym for "class." The isotype of an antibody (e.g., IgA or IgG) is determined by the constant region of its heavy chain.

Lc: Light chain protein of the antibody molecule.

Leukocytes: A generic term that includes all of the different kinds of white blood cells.

Ligand: A molecule that binds to a receptor (e.g., the Fas ligand binds to the Fas receptor protein on the surface of a cell).

Ligate: Bind to. When a receptor has bound its ligand, the receptor is said to be "ligated."

Lipopolysaccharide (LPS): A component of many bacterial cell walls that serves as a "danger signal" for the innate system.

Lymph: The liquid that "leaks" out of blood vessels into the tissues.

Lymphocyte: The generic term for a B cell or a T cell.

Lymphoid follicle: A region of a secondary lymphoid organ that contains follicular dendritic cells embedded in a sea of B cells.

M cell: A cell that crowns a Peyer's patch, and which specializes in sampling antigen from the intestine.

MALT: Mucosal associated lymphoid tissues. Secondary lymphoid organs that are associated with mucosa (e.g., Peyer's patches and tonsils).

Medullary thymic epithelial cell: A cell in the medulla of the thymus which expresses tissue-specific self antigens, and which takes part in the examination of T cells for tolerance of self (negative selection).

Memory effector T cells: Memory T cells that lie dormant in the tissues until an enemy attacks again.

MHC proteins: Proteins encoded by the major histocompatibility complex (the region of a chromosome that includes a "complex" of genes involved in antigen presentation).

MHC restriction: Survival in the thymus is "restricted" to T cells whose receptors recognize antigen presented by MHC molecules.

Microbe: A generic term that includes bacteria and viruses.

Monocytes: White blood cells that are the precursors of macrophages or dendritic cells.

Mucosa: The tissues and associated mucus that protect exposed surfaces such as the gastrointestinal and respiratory tracts.

Naive lymphocytes: B or T cells which never have been activated.

Natural regulatory T cells (nTregs): CD4$^+$ T cells that are selected in the thymus and which negatively regulate the immune response by interfering with the activation of self-reactive T cells in the secondary lymphoid organs.

Necrosis: Cell death, typically caused by burns or other trauma. This type of cell death (as opposed to apoptotic cell death) usually results in the contents of the cell being dumped into the tissues. This can cause tissue damage.

Negative selection: Synonym for "central tolerance induction." The selection of T cells whose receptors do not recognize MHC–self peptide complexes in the thymus.

NK cell: Natural killer cell. A player on the innate system team.

Oncogene: A mutated proto-oncogene which encodes a protein that can cause cells to proliferate inappropriately.

Opsonize: "Decorate" with fragments of complement proteins or with antibodies.

Pathogen: A disease-causing agent (e.g., a bacterium or a virus).

Peptide: A small fragment of a protein, usually only tens of amino acids in length.

Peripheral tolerance: The result of mechanisms that induce self tolerance outside the thymus.

Phagocytes: Cells such as macrophages and neutrophils that engulf (phagocytose) invaders.

Plasma B cells: Short-lived plasma B cells produce a large burst of antibodies in response to an attack and die. Long-lived plasma B cells make more modest amounts of antibodies that confer long-term protection.

Positive selection: Synonym for "MHC restriction."

Primary lymphoid organs: The thymus and the bone marrow.

Proliferate: Increase in number. A cell proliferates by dividing into two daughter cells, which can divide again to give four cells, and so on. Cellular reproduction.

Proteasome: A multi-protein complex in the cell that chops proteins up into small pieces.

Proto-oncogene: A gene which, if mutated, can become an oncogene.

Receptor editing: The process by which a B cell, whose receptors recognize a self antigen, gets a "second chance" to rearrange its receptors and avoid deletion in the bone marrow.

Secondary lymphoid organs: Organs such as lymph nodes, Peyer's patches, and the spleen where activation of naive B and T cells takes place.

Secrete: Export out of the cell (e.g., cytokines are secreted by the T cells that produce them, and B cells secrete antibodies).

TCR: T cell receptor.

Th: Helper T cell.

Thymic dendritic cell: A starfish-shaped cell located in the medulla of the thymus which administers the exam for tolerance of self (negative selection) to T cells.

TNF: Tumor necrosis factor. A cytokine secreted mainly by macrophages and helper T cells.

Tolerance of self: Not viewing self as an attacker which should be targeted for destruction.

Tolerize: To make a B cell or T cell tolerant of our self antigens.

Toll-like receptors: Receptor molecules found either on the surface of cells or inside cells. These receptors have evolved to recognize the signatures of common invaders and to generate signals which alert the immune system to danger.

Tumor suppressor protein: A protein which is part of a control system within a cell that safeguards against inappropriate cell proliferation.

Virgin (naive) lymphocytes: B or T cells which never have been activated.

Index

How the Immune System Works, Fourth Edition. Lauren Sompayrac. © 2012 John Wiley & Sons, Ltd. Published 2012 by John Wiley & Sons, Ltd.